T0073851

YouthSites

YouthSites

HISTORIES OF CREATIVITY, CARE, AND LEARNING IN THE CITY

Stuart R. Poyntz, Julian Sefton-Green, and
Heather Fitzsimmons Frey

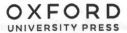

OXFORD
UNIVERSITY PRESS

OXFORD
UNIVERSITY PRESS

Oxford University Press is a department of the University of Oxford. It furthers
the University's objective of excellence in research, scholarship, and education
by publishing worldwide. Oxford is a registered trade mark of Oxford University
Press in the UK and certain other countries.

Published in the United States of America by Oxford University Press
198 Madison Avenue, New York, NY 10016, United States of America.

© Oxford University Press 2023

Library of Congress Cataloging-in-Publication Data
Names: Poyntz, Stuart R., author. | Sefton-Green, Julian, author. |
Fitzsimmons Frey, Heather, author.
Title: YouthSites : histories of creativity, care, and learning in the city /
Stuart R. Poyntz, Julian Sefton-Green, and Heather Fitzsimmons Frey.
Description: New York : Oxford University Press, [2023] |
Includes bibliographical references and index. |
Identifiers: LCCN 2022053510 (print) | LCCN 2022053511 (ebook) |
ISBN 9780197555491 (Hardback) | ISBN 9780197555514 (epub) | ISBN 9780197555521
Subjects: LCSH: Non-formal education. | Alternative education.
Classification: LCC LC45.3.P69 2023 (print) | LCC LC45.3 (ebook) |
DDC 371.04—dc23/eng/20230110
LC record available at https://lccn.loc.gov/2022053510
LC ebook record available at https://lccn.loc.gov/2022053511

DOI: 10.1093/oso/9780197555491.001.0001

Printed by Integrated Books International, United States of America

CONTENTS

CONTENTS

LIST OF ILLUSTRATIONS

Figures

Table

ACKNOWLEDGMENTS

The idea for this book germinated in 2013 when Stuart Poyntz, Michael Hoechsmann, and Julian Sefton-Green first met as a result of Stuart and Michael's Social Sciences and Humanities Research Council of Canada (SSHRC)-funded, Youth Digital Media Ecologies grant exploring the ecology of youth provision in Vancouver and Toronto, Canada. Stuart subsequently led a successful application for a larger SSHRC-funded project, Networks of Non-Formal Learning, which commenced in 2015. Our first thanks go to the SSHRC and the fraternal collegiality of Michael Hoechsmann, with whom we worked on the project from 2014 to 2019. His experience, calm, and insights have been with us every step of the way. The team expanded over the period significantly to include Heather Fitzsimmons Frey, and the three of us have collaborated on the book as joint authors. Despite enormous distances (Julian moved from London to Melbourne in 2017) and pandemic restrictions, we have managed to work as a team bringing together the research presented in this book. We credit each other's skills, patience, and support throughout the years.

Many people have helped us along the way. These include research assistants and of course the leaders and workers at the organizations we have studied. Sometimes these people are named, and so in that way, we credit their participation; in other instances, we thank the workers and administrators who supported our aims in bringing to light the important work these organizations do with and for young people in Vancouver, Toronto, and London.

Before listing the various organizations and individuals who helped us along the way, we note the special contribution of Rebecca (Becky) Coles, based in the United Kingdom, who not only carried out much of the fieldwork in London but also worked collectively with us designing and developing the research processes that enabled us to map the organizations across both countries. Equally crucial thanks go to Alysha Bains, who worked both in Vancouver and on the project more generally as a PhD scholar at Simon Fraser University. We also thank Elesha May Daley, Madison Byblow, Averie MacDonald, Melissa Fellin, and iowyth hezel ulthiin (formerly Cassandra Witteman) for their contributions to the research.

We thank the following for their significant help: in Vancouver, Elaine Carol (Miscellaneous Productions), Gurp Sian (South Asian Arts), Deblekha Guin (Access to Media Education Society), Venay Feldon, Tammy Bannister and Maria Cecelia Sab (Reel2Real International Film Festival for Youth), Mark Vonesch (Reel Youth), Corin Brown, Patti Fraser, Liz Schulze, and Pia Massie; in Toronto, Randell Adjei (RISE Edutainment), Jason Samilski (CUE), Jen Fabico (Scarborough Arts),

Marlene McKintosh and Lensa Simesso Denga (Urban Arts), Craig Morrison and Lauren Hortie (Oasis Skateboard Factory), Phyllis Novak and Sue Cohen (SKETCH), Nikki Shaffeeullah and Rachel Penny (The Artists Mentoring Youth [AMY] Project), Michael Prosserman (Unity Charity), Kate Welsh (AMY board chair), Karen Emerson (Children's Peace Theatre), Dorothy Ann Manuel and Caroline Mangosing (Kapisanan), Dwayne Dixon (Nia), Angola Murdoch (Talk to Youth Lately), Adonis Huggins (Regent Park), Rita Davies, and Loree Lawrence; in London, Paul Owens and Callum Lee (BOP Consulting), Graham Hitchen, Denise Stanley, and Tom Campbell. Special thanks also go to Celia Greenwood, Nii Sackey, Deborah Beswick, Steve Shaw, and Camille Curtis y van Dyke. In Australia, thanks to Navid Sabet and Natalie Hendry.

We are deeply grateful for hundreds of participants and past participants, facilitators, artists, and mentors who contributed to our research in countless ways.

Finally, we thank Dawn Rushen for her help in preparing the manuscript and the team at Oxford University Press (OUP), including the anonymous reviewers used by OUP, for their support in making this book happen.

In Canada, many academics are choosing to offer a land acknowledgement. YouthSites is a multisite project, and members of our team have been privileged to work as guests on multiple territories, and through virtual space. We acknowledge the lands in the spaces we now call Toronto and Vancouver that nurture the artists, youth, and arts organizations we discuss in this book. Tkaronto (Toronto) is Dish with One Spoon and Two Row Wampum Territory of many nations, including the Mississaugas of the Credit, the Haudenosaunee Confederacy, the Huron-Wendat, and the Seneca. K'emk'emlay (Vancouver) is on the unceded territories of the Coast Salish peoples of the xʷməθkwəy̓əm (Musqueam), Skwxwú7mesh (Squamish), and Səlílwətaɬ (Tsleil-Waututh) Nations. Both these cities are now home to many diverse First Nations, Inuit, and Métis peoples from across Turtle Island, who are caretakers past, present, and future.

In addition, we acknowledge that Heather now works in Treaty 6 Territory amiskwaciwâskahikan / ⊲⌐ᒃ·⌐ᐧᖬᖚᐊᑲᑉ (Edmonton), which many First Nations, Inuit, and Métis people call home today. Significant as a gathering and trading place since time immemorial, traditional caretakers in Treaty 6 include ᑐᖚᐊᐳᐤ ⊲ᐣᑭᐩ nêhiyawak (Cree), Tsuu T'ina (Blackfoot), Dene, and Métis, as well as Ojibway/Saulteaux/Anishinaabe and Kanien'kehá: ka (Mohawk) Nations. For much of our work on this book, Julian was present at Deakin University in Melbourne, Australia, where the Wurndjeri people of the Kulin nations are the Traditional Owners of the land.

Finally, we acknowledge the caretakers of many lands, both near and far, whose territories support the infrastructures that make gathering in virtual space possible. In particular, we extend our thanks to the Muwekma Ohlone tribal nation, whose traditional territories accommodate Zoom's headquarters in Palo Alto, California. We are grateful to gather and work on these lands and in virtual space, and pay our respects to the caretakers and Elders, past, present, and future.

ABOUT THE AUTHORS

Stuart R. Poyntz is Professor and Director of the School of Communication and a Director of the Community Engaged Research Initiative at Simon Fraser University. He has been a Visiting Scholar at Queensland University of Technology, Griffith University, Hong Kong Baptist University, and the University of British Columbia, and he was President of the Association for Research in Cultures of Young People from 2012 to 2017. From 1996 to 2003, he was Director of Education at The Cinémathèque, Western Canada's leading film institute, where he led a series of film and media education and production programs and wrote and co-produced the Knowledge Network's *Depth of Field* television series for educators. He has since published four books, numerous journal articles and book chapters, and has been invited to speak at universities and with public school educators in China, Australia, the United Kingdom, Hong Kong, South Korea, and Canada.

Julian Sefton-Green is Professor of New Media Education at Deakin University, Melbourne, Australia. He has held positions at the Department of Media & Communication, London School of Economics & Political Science and at the University of Oslo. In a varied career including high school teaching, teacher education, and being an independent scholar, he has been the Head of Media Arts and Education at WAC Performing Arts and Media College, a center for informal training and education, where he directed a range of digital media activities for young people and coordinated training for media artists and teachers. He has researched and written widely on many aspects of media education, new technologies, creativity, digital cultures, and informal learning and has authored, co-authored, or edited 20 books and has spoken at more than 50 conferences in approximately 20 different countries. https://julianseftongr een.net

Heather Fitzsimmons Frey is an Assistant Professor of Arts and Cultural Management at MacEwan University in Edmonton and holds a PhD in Drama, Theatre, and Performance Studies from the University of Toronto. Using archives, qualitative research methods such as interviews and focus groups, performance-based historiography, and practice-based creative methodologies, her research focuses on the arts and cultural sector and young people, in both historical and contemporary contexts. Prior to working in the sector, she was a public high school teacher, and for 6 years she was volunteer staff and eventually director for the youth-run Alberta-based Seminar on the United Nations and International Affairs; subsequently, she served on the board for many years. Her research is published in diverse journals and books, including *Girlhood Studies*, *Jeunesse*, *Journal of Childhood Studies*, *Performance Research*, *Theatre Research in Canada / Recherches Théâtrales au Canada*, and *Theatre Research International*.

1

A History of Changing Places for Learning, Creativity, and Care in the City

Introduction

This is a book about a sector that is not recognized as such, organizations that do not like being institutionalized, forms of education that exist outside the mainstream curriculum, types of aesthetic expression that are often unrecognized, visions of civic participation that run against the grain, and opportunities for socially marginalized young people who are frequently denied them. And yet, it is also a book about established, fairly well resourced projects and activities that are often evaluated and monitored by local authorities at the city level or even the nation state; the projects often fit within a complex network of routes for young people across learning institutions in the city, and they are frequently the result of high-profile, highly public initiatives, branding, and advocacy.

The subject of this book is difficult to name. Essentially, we set out to study what, in the United Kingdom, has been called "the non-formal learning sector," referring to a raft of organizations that offer young people, frequently from low-income families, opportunities to participate, learn about, and possibly be trained in a range of performing and creative arts. These organizations do not go by any single name, although they do build on a shared history in community arts (from the 1960s) or youth arts (from the 1970s) or even arts-led youth provision (an even older form of pre–World War II welfare provision). The naming problem was made acute by the fact that we set out to research these organizations in two countries—Canada and the United Kingdom—and specifically in three cities: London, Toronto, and Vancouver. The different powers accorded to central authorities in both countries, with the distinction in Canada between federal and province not being entirely mirrored by the United Kingdom's distinction between national and local authority, makes the problem of definition more complex because how these organizations are funded also tends to define them.

YouthSites. Stuart R. Poyntz, Julian Sefton-Green, and Heather Fitzsimmons Frey, Oxford University Press.
© Oxford University Press 2023. DOI: 10.1093/oso/9780197555491.003.0001

As will become apparent at different stages throughout the book, we have all had different direct experience of working with these organizations, and so came to the project with a sense of shared practices and traditions, systems, and structures that seemed to make the idea of a common phenomenon coherent and logical. There is evidence of out-of-school, youth-focused state and independently run organizations offering media and arts activities for young people across many cities throughout the world. In some cases, this has been approached from the point of view of supplementary or complementary forms of education that have grown up around "mainstream" provision, and it has been termed "a shadow education system" (Bray, 2009). In other cases, the key object of enquiry has been the neighborhood and community setting and its relationship to the production of locally meaningful art (Crehan, 2011). In some circumstances, attention has been given to how young people themselves have been organized and/or organize themselves as a way of providing forms of institutional status to support their interests (Kirshner, 2015). In yet other circumstances, the attention has been on provision for displaced and marginalized youth with an interest in projects that emphasize belonging and reengagement (DeLuca et al., 2016). And there are also a whole raft of studies examining forms of alternative pedagogy and creative practices that stem from an attention to these original social and learning spaces, ranging from photography in London in the 1980s to online radio in Oakland, California, in the second decade of the 21st century, or even graffiti and hip-hop projects in Medellin, Colombia (Brough, 2020; Dewdney & Lister, 1988; Soep & Chavez, 2010).

There has been a range of social policy, youth, education, and arts scholarship that has systematically paid attention to the ingenuity and diversity of locally based organizations that have often been led by remarkable individuals working in difficult and challenging circumstances in cities throughout the world. Yet, despite this shared history, and despite a shared sense of practices, activities, values, and even possibly belief in similar outcomes, there have been remarkably few studies of what we want to think of as a sector or organizational type in any one country let alone international comparisons (Sefton-Green & Erstad, 2018).

This is primarily because the accounts of these organizations have been offered from one of the analytic perspectives described above. Thus, scholars of education are interested in out-of-school learning, scholars of youth in youth activism, scholars of art in community art, and so forth. Although we examine the systemic and structural nature of these organizations, and throughout this book show that although they may stem from single-issue organizations, they often mutate to meet a variety of interests and concerns in practice, we note this has not been the object of previous scholarship. We think this is an omission that deserves correction. More than that, we argue here that paying attention to the ebb and flow of organizations that frequently rise and fall more than the formal sectors of education or arts or youth work (categories that are frequently institutionalized and receive consistent revenue funding) brings out of the shadows a whole set of practices, entrepreneurial activity, social enterprises, and interlinked youth education networks, and thus articulates a distinct historical narrative about provision for and the production of youth since the 1990s.

We set out to examine groups of organizations in the three cities over three decades: the 1990s, 2000s, and 2010s. We wanted to pay attention to the shifts in funding, setup, and delivery in these organizations or the "non-formal learning sector," as we term it, because they shed light on key absences, alternatives to their comparator organizations in the mainstream, and this form of social rebalancing itself hints at deeper structural recalibration within the matrix of institutions and sectors that traditionally comprise welfare provision in the two countries. Although the roots of the organizations lie in forms of community organizing and, indeed, community arts as much as they do in state-mandated youth provision (and in Canada this has an inflection toward serving Indigenous youth just as in London it hints at an equality of provision for young people from minority ethnic backgrounds), since 1990 we have witnessed significant restructuring of state institutions at all levels. A key argument is that our sector that is not a sector in formal bureaucratic terms exemplifies ways that the neoliberal state has attempted to manage "educational failure" and "troublesome youth" through an appeal to forms of a "creative future."

Our focus on these organizations thus brings together a wide range of interests and concerns about the ways in which education is imagined, youth are served, and creativity (the arts) is harnessed by the modern state—particularly working at the city level. The lack of formal definition as an economic or administrative sector (in the ways that "the arts" or "education" are now accepted common sense) only serves to support our thesis that the sector has acted as an extraordinary kind of valve or coping mechanism—perhaps the cynics might say, even as a mop—to contain and control other kinds of social injustice and inequality as young people, especially from low-income families, have found their options and opportunities circumscribed in ever more unequal societies (Dorling, 2011; Wilkinson & Pickett, 2010).

Yet, our interest was stimulated and engaged by the extraordinary imagination, drive, care, love, and practical ingenuity demonstrated by these organizations as they have worked with young people in challenging circumstances in the three cities since 1990. For all the ways that we argue that changing state regimes tried to pull levers and push buttons in order to contain and control the very young people who, it could be argued, they have hitherto failed, we also want to represent—in the sense of argue for—the diverse ways that these organizations have inspired, led, and changed the lives of youth since 1990. Our interest in the idea of sectors and institutions does not stand in the way of examining how hybrid forms of organization mutated and, less commonly, stayed constant to the core principles of social justice. This balance between the wider demands of the state and how they were and are interpreted and negotiated at individual, aesthetic, pedagogic, and organizational levels lies at the heart of our ambition to analyze these organizations.

At the beginning of our project, we came up with the term "YouthSites"—places for young people as well as spaces where they are seen and made visible. Because the "non-formal learning sector" is both a bit of a mouthful and perhaps overemphasizes the side of these organizations that interfaces with education, we use the term YouthSites alongside the term non-formal learning sector because for all of our conviction that together these organizations do comprise a sector in a bureaucratic sense, it appears only to be one seen by scholars, practitioners, young people, and their families rather than by society at large.

The subject of this book, then, is the organizations themselves—their histories, the people, their practices, their impacts, and what wider social purpose they are seen to achieve. Collectively, we think they comprise a kind of administrative sector, in the sense of publicly funded institutions working to fulfill a conventional social remit, either at national or city level. The idea of a sector and even, at times, the curiously made-up nature of these organizations' institutional status also means that as an object of enquiry, they exist on the boundaries. Although the organizations themselves are discrete phenomena and comprise a series of activities in relationship to young people, practitioners (social work, youth work, and the arts), funding agencies, published reports, and so on, in definitional terms they are also best understood as what they are not (Sefton-Green, 2013). They are like schools but not schools, they espouse creative production but have no credentials, they are homes for many young people and yet they are transitory. This sense of our subject, our organizations, being constructed on the boundaries of conventional social analysis is central to the purpose of this book, but it presents us with a series of scholarly challenges as we try to disentangle all the various contexts, themes, and histories that have gone into these organizations and that continue to sustain their activities at the margins.

Overview of Contexts, Themes, and Histories

We begin with an anatomy of an organization, not that we think that any one organization can stand for all of them, but to give some sense of the uniqueness of how it works and in particular to help readers get a feel for the quality of the experience that animated our research. We then offer a brief overview of the size and scope of "the sector," or at least how some understanding of the aggregate of these organizations contributes to the notion of a discrete "field" of action. That term is, of course, taken from Bourdieu (1990, 1993), and we prefigure some of the debate about what it means to talk about these organizations working as a sector or field and their relationship to funding.

The question of funding raises the challenge of how these organizations and their work are commissioned—setting aside the entrepreneurial drive of their leaders—and thus the role they play in fulfilling a range of social, educational, and arts policy objectives. We have attempted to study these organizations over a

30-year period that has seen the retrenchment of welfare, the deployment of new forms of governance, and, of course, the effects of the globalizing economic order known as neoliberalism. The relationship between the institutional nature of these organizations and their aggregate impact and the changing role of the neoliberal state constitutes our third section.

As we have already argued, these organizations work at the intersection of the more established fields of education, arts (community arts in particular), and urban youth provision. The history of each of these sectors, their significant changes over the time period of our research, and indeed, the ways that their scope of operations has changed, form the content of subsequent sections. The final section introduces questions around our methods, the choice of the three cities and the timescale we chose to investigate, and this leads into an outline of the book as a whole, with particular attention to how we constructed our research as both a historical and an international comparison. We end this introductory chapter by reiterating the significance and importance of the organizations in this sector as a field of study.

Regent Park Focus Youth Media Arts Centre: Anatomy of a YouthSite

When Adonis Huggins was an early hire at the Regent Park Focus Youth Media Arts Centre in 1990, the neighborhood of Regent Park was a run-down, inner-city area of Toronto, Canada, with dense public housing and sporadic public concerns around young people's vulnerability to drugs, alcohol, and youth violence. A young 14-year-old boy, Benji Haywood, had been found dead in Lake Ontario, and the city's response was to set up Focus community programs to offer young people structured and organized forms of participation to intervene in what was seen as a spiral of deprivation. Huggins himself came from a background in community theater, and as a young Black man who has grown up in Toronto's inner city, he had a political investment in supporting forms of Black culture and minority arts. He himself had attended a community center in the Kensington Market area run by the Anglican Church.

From the very beginning in the early 1990s, Huggins articulated a clear set of principles for engaging young people using the arts with the belief that civic participation needed to be driven by young people themselves, that the content should come from them and their peer cultures. He focused on video and encouraged young people to make socially engaged documentary investigations about matters of interest to them in their community. In a pre-internet age, the challenge was to find ways of distribution for these films in the form of a television channel so that young people's voices and concerns could be equally represented in the public sphere.

Nearly 30 years later, the same vision, the same focus, and the same set of practices animate the work of Regent Park Focus. Although the numbers of young people who attend each year are not incredibly high—approximately 200 young people between ages 14 and 29 years attended in 2015, for example—the young people themselves make a substantial commitment to the creative and civic opportunities offered by Regent Park Focus. Sometimes they stay for 1 year but frequently for up to 5 years and often even beyond that as the organization has a commitment to supporting and developing young people to become members of staff who work as mentors, filmmakers, and tutors alongside other artists who are employed on short-term grants. The young people themselves are positioned as leaders and directors of the creative projects, whereas more senior artists take on a more supportive role throughout the production process.

Huggins has continued to hustle and has a model of institutional development in which he strings one grant onto another in order to make things happen. The persistence and commitment of the young people offer a form of continuity and institutional stability so that projects and expertise in practice can continue to grow. The relatively small-scale focus of the organization has continued to reflect community concerns and the urgency and relevance of community-based art. Board members and artists tend to be local, with a history of community-based activism across Toronto. The young people are racially diverse, and at different times through the organization's history it has set out to engage, for example, South Asian youth or Indigenous youth in a deliberate attempt to involve discrete and particular political trajectories in its work.

The media ecology that spawned Regent Park Focus with its interest in voice and the difficulty of distributing media by and for the community has, of course, radically transformed since 1995, and nowadays it offers multimedia programs (free at the point of use) in radio, video, audio arts, photography, music, magazine, and new media, as well as dedicated programs for "Divas" deliberately targeting and engaging young women. The concern with distribution and the development of a local community television channel, to act as a community focus, has, of course, been enabled by the growth of the internet, but nevertheless, the attention to bringing young people together physically to work on collective projects and to the development of meaningful forms of public distribution and commentary about local issues remains central.

The language used in grant applications to profile the organization talks of "culturally marginalized diverse youth" and consistently and repeatedly emphasizes values of community and belonging. The power to document lives at the margins, but also to engage with politicians and other civil authorities such as the police, gives the work of the organization energy and purpose.

Regent Park Focus' activities usually take place after school every weekday but extend into a summer camp, and they frequently involve partnering with more established Toronto organizations, such as the Royal Ontario Museum or Toronto Public Health. Small-scale local funding and relationships with city-based organizations enable a range of project funding to drive a continuous raft of activities. Outreach project work with schools and other community organizations drives recruitment and projects.

More recently, the billion-dollar redevelopment of the neighborhood of Regent Park has taken the organization with it in terms of expanding spaces, activities, and profile. The organization negotiated a move to a more institutional space as part of its own growth, but the new space is provided virtually free (rent is CA$2 per year), even if operating expenses to support this level of resourcing take up approximately CA$40,000 a year from an annual budget of approximately CA$250,000.[1] In this context, Regent Park Focus has continued to rely on its history with local people to sustain its values in a complex period of technological change, intense gentrification in Toronto, and changes in the local community.

The Non-Formal Learning Sector in London

Regent Park Focus has quite a long history in the lives of a particular community. Although there is no doubt that its effect on many young people's lives can be ascribed to the entrepreneurial energy of its staff, and especially its founder, its ethos and practices are not only found elsewhere throughout Toronto but also exist in many cities throughout the world. Although organizations such as Regent Park Focus are often appreciated for their singularity, they do, in fact, exemplify both an institutional type and structure, and they form part of a strata of state and privately funded organizations that link together discrete zones of youth activity and concern. In the United Kingdom, this is known as the "voluntary sector"; in the United States, it is called the "not-for-profit sector." In some places throughout the world, the terminology of "nongovernmental organization" is used.

A key aim of this book is to explicate what it might mean to consider the ways that youth-oriented education, community, and arts practices have evolved from initiatives and projects into organizations and, indeed, institutions that together comprise a form of administrative bureaucratic sectoral identity. To begin this process, we describe the scope and range of these organizations operating in London since 1990 (and, to an extent, we could have told a similar story in Toronto or Vancouver) to give readers unfamiliar with this "sector" a sense of reach, permanence, turnover, and practice. We return to the metaphor of "institutional evolution" (here beginning with community-based social practices and leading to forms of business incorporation, capital investment, and institutional habitus, as described in the history of Regent Park Focus) throughout this book because such a process, we argue, has created the condition for its own destruction as much as it has enabled success. In addition, we challenge the teleology of evolution implicit in the conceptual nature of institutionalization.

Following a 2002 inquiry into how best to support the growth of London's creative industries led by the Mayor of London, the London Development Agency (LDA; at that time, the Mayor's agency responsible for economic growth) set up the Supporting Talent to Enterprise Programme (STEP) enquiry into the non-formal learning sector for the creative industries in London (Hitchins et al., 2014). The study found 250 organizations working with more than 35,000 learners, of whom 58% were from Black and minority ethnic backgrounds, 47% lived locally, and 11% had a disability. The 2004 report effectively argued that together, what it called the STEP organizations, or non-formal learning sector, comprised the size and reach of a good-sized university offering learning experiences throughout London, even though many of the organizations might originally view themselves more in terms of their social and community impact. As an agency responsible for economic growth, the LDA was interested in the organizations' industry links and the progression routes in place for learners. Through its research, it sought recognition and credibility for the sector, and it explored how it could be more strategically led, its funding stabilized, and how industry might recognize qualifications achieved through non-formal arts groups (Burns Owens Partnership & Stanley, 2004). Even in 2004, however, 42% of funding received by the organizations had to be renewed annually, leaving the sector, even at the height of its recognition, fragile and unable to plan for the long term (Burns Owens Partnership & Stanley, 2004).

Indeed, we found a shift in funding sources over a 30-year period. In 1995, the largest proportion of funding came from local public sources, many local councils (London is divided into 32 democratically accountable local authorities). By 2005, the largest proportion of funding came from national public sources, such as the Arts Council England, but by 2015 third-sector or self-generated income (e.g., from renting space) had become the most significant funding source. Individual organizations varied dramatically in terms of their size and scope, although this is difficult to measure (as we discuss in Chapter 2) due to the fact that some organizations were projects attached to larger national bodies, and in many cases, freelance staff made it difficult to get a sense of scale from examining core personnel costs. Some organizations have up to 1,000 young people a week coming through their doors; others only 25.

In general, the 250 organizations, some of which had been founded in the late 1970s and some of which have had very short "lives," focused on discrete art forms: music and music production, dance, drama, and the spoken word, as well as media. Some specialized in specific media, such as Regent Park Focus center's focus on video; others were more generic. If art form focus, or funding, varied, what these organizations have in common was a focus on young people targeted on the basis of ethnicity, social disadvantage, or disengagement or exclusion from education, and also on the basis of gender, disability or illness, being vulnerable, being "at risk," unemployment, involvement in crime, or radicalization. In Canada, indigeneity also provided a key focus. The London organizations tended to cluster around four types with regard to examining their aims and purpose: (a) a "youth arts" focus on young people and their well-being and preparation for adult life; (b) an "art form or creative industry interests" aimed at tying social and individual outcomes to artistic ones—that is, developing art form expertise and expanding access to that art form for excluded groups; (c) more explicit "arts education and vocational training" with a focus on training artists and workers for the creative industry; and (d) as a resource to support the creation of youth culture—original songs, videos, poetry, and dances—to scaffold young people's exploration of ideas, aesthetics, identity, and a sense of their own voices.

Some of the organizations comprising this non-formal learning sector also offered outreach work in schools, professional venues, touring, training for adults, and apprenticeship in the creative industries. There seemed to be three main ways the organizations structured their work with young people. First were stand-alone workshops, often taking place during a school term or semester, including on-going weekly classes and/or holiday programs. If classes took place in school time, they recruited from young people who had been excluded from formal education or who were, at that time, beyond a statutory age to attend school. Second were targeted projects via a contract or commission by local authority or another organization. This model derived funding from targeted initiatives—for example, contracts for short breaks for children and young people with disabilities or programs for young people at risk through specific referral from social services. Third were activities offering specific and bespoke courses or apprenticeships, such as a 10-week training program for 14- to 25-year-olds interested in events management.

Very few organizations offered qualifications in 1995, but by 2005, forms of vocational qualifications were on offer. By 2015, it was much more common for organizations to offer forms of accreditation that might involve recognition of participation but might also involve certification by attainment. We return to the issue of micro-credentialing and the debates around forms of vocational (often industry-led) certification and the relationship of both practices to attainment, as it is understood as an outcome of the formal education system throughout this book.

Where activities took place was, and is, important. Some organizations had been gifted buildings through National Lottery–funded sources, and these were often used as ways of mitigating financial loss and deriving income. However, renting the local hall was often where many of these organizations had started out. The relationship between gentrification and spiraling property prices in London had an impact both on where these organizations had initially started and on where they were forced to move due to rising costs—this was especially an issue as marginalized youth were being pushed from the inner to the outer fringes of the city over the 30-year period.

One key feature of a governmental sector is the equal treatment of institutions (e.g., hospitals or schools). However, a distinguishing feature of this sector is the way that the organizations within it were often in competition with each other and frequently rivals in securing finite revenue from finite grant sources. The fact that they ended up developing similar morphological characteristics perhaps reveals more about the ways that their origins derived from education, arts, or youth practices as much as parallel adaptations to the same funding ecologies. Nevertheless, as the 2004 STEP report maintained (Burns Owens Partnership &

Stanley, 2004), these organizations worked in parallel, often in relationship with similar formal sectors (e.g., in one local authority, several organizations might support young people who attended the schools in that area); they worked similarly in relationship with top-down funding streams; and they offered forms of very similar structural organization and participation. In that sense, they represent a continuous segment of youth-focused institutions that have always existed in large cities—certainly in the United Kingdom and Canada, but also in Europe, the United States, and Australia—during the past 50–60 years, even if their presence as a sector has rarely been registered by scholars and policymakers for youth, education, and the arts.

The Neoliberal State

Our attention to organizational form, arts, and educational practices, the processes of institutionalization, and indeed, the way that when aggregated we seemed to be looking at a much broader process of bureaucratic structure, suggested to us that the non-formal learning sector actually offers a unique lens to examine the ways that the neoliberal state works. Although the next two chapters describe in much more detail ways in which the operation of these organizations and their sector has changed since 1990, even the very brief outline above about changes in funding, accreditation, and the changing relationship to property shows how new kinds of contemporary civic institution have emerged in concert with the transformation of traditional welfare provision.

As we describe, the roots of the non-formal learning sector lie in forms of community art, alternative education, and youth services. All three of these areas have their origins in 20th-century movements and clearly form part of the landscape of provision available in both Canada and the United Kingdom as part of post–World War II settlements. The emergence in the 1980s of the new global political order of neoliberalism (D. Harvey, 2007, 2011) led to both the retrenchment and an expansion of the ways that the state delivered these kinds of provision. As is well known, broad trends in national politics in both the United Kingdom and Canada during this period saw the privatization and marketization of previously state-controlled welfare provision as social mobility decreased, social inequality increased, and centralized government dispersed. We draw attention to three aspects of this larger process, which, we argue, saw the sector drive change as much as it could be said to reflect the restructuring of private and public capital.

A key plank of the neoliberal rhetoric is to reduce the power and reach of the state in favor of the market. In both Canada and the United Kingdom, private out-of-school arts and learning activities have always sustained a small market where middle-class families have traditionally purchased music, drama, or dance lessons as part of a general enrichment, using after-school activities to supplement the curriculum (Lareau, 2011). The growth of youth and community arts, particularly when supported through grants from left-leaning progressive city authorities, such as the Greater London Council in the 1980s, helped expand this private market, creating opportunities for young people who had typically been denied privileged access. By the mid-1990s, local authority funding, which effectively tied the service to the funder as a revenue-client, began to be mixed with other forms of procurement such as philanthropic funds, centralized government competitive grants, and, in the United Kingdom, the availability of European money. Further sources of income from private foundations changed the model of centrally driven service delivery to one of competitive tender. Organizations had to apply for, and would live or die by their success in attaining, open grants.

The growth of the non-formal learning sector as a mix of organizations and/or projects is directly attributable to these changes in funding arrangements, which themselves derive from an attempt to develop a market-driven model of service delivery. First, money for these services was now coming not just from the state but also from a range of sources (charities and, later, private foundations). Second, emphasis shifted from continuing to support institutions toward outcomes-driven projects. Rather than just supporting an institution because it always worked with young people in a particular area, the focus now shifted toward delivering projects that met specific outcomes—for example, reaching X number of young people from Y minority ethnic group. Such a changing regime supported the growth of new organizations and shifted attention away from traditional institutional expertise toward the capability of projects to comply with new kinds of regulatory schemes. In most cases, this meant that success was determined by a new kind of regulatory mechanism, from the growth of monitoring and evaluation industries to simple numerical compliance. The organizations thus emerged into a culture of bid rhetoric (or being able to describe and advocate for their work in competitive terms) and evaluation rhetoric (being able to demonstrate measures as required by the new regulatory state).

A further implication of this change in the relationship between state, institutions, procurement, and compliance has been evident in the changing nature of governance and self-governance over the period. Several scholars have noted that whereas in the past the power of the state was visible and explicit, the current era is characterized by forms of increasingly internalized self-regulation (Rose, 1999). Individuals are now held responsible for their life course in ways that social structure may previously have taken responsibility for them. This has meant not only a growth in the lifelong learning agenda (Field, 2006, 2008) as people are required to pick up forms of accreditation to qualify them for increasingly precarious and competitive employment prospects but also responsibility for social success is being increasingly devolved through layers of government, from the center outwards. Again, the organizations can be seen to be playing a part in this recalibration of responsibility. First, they became liable for ensuring the success of the marginalized youth they served, and this tended to mean financial risks for the organizations and staff involved. Second, they became new places for young people themselves to discharge the responsibilities of managing their own learning and training. They thus embodied and inculcated new disciplines of what has been called the "responsibilization of governance."

The second key area in which we can see the organizations developing in response to the changing role of the state is in relationship to property speculation and gentrification. The period of time we studied has witnessed significant changes in the demographic and material composition of the inner city. In general, across all of the three cities, we have seen a move from a deprived inner city, often disproportionately populated by people of color, and from marginalized communities toward the process of property speculation, a dramatic increase in rents, and, eventually, the dispossession of the original inhabitants of these communities toward the outer suburbs. Many of the organizations began in the inner city, working with what were then local communities, but now they often serve young people who have to travel across the city to reach them. Public support for buildings and capital investment has supported the process of gentrification, thus frequently leading to changes in circumstances, which has meant that the organizations can no longer afford to inhabit the properties they were granted to achieve their purposes.

This symbiotic relationship the organizations have with their locale brings us to the third key theme in the ways that the modern state now relates to its population, which is specifically around the place of youth in the city—and here the use of ciphers such as the phrase "urban youth" often stands for what are perceived to be troublesome or marginalized communities—mainly, in our context, meaning young people of color. The management of troublesome youth has long been a concern of contemporary post-war societies in terms of circumscribing visibility and presence, especially with regard to policing public spaces in the city (and hence, increasingly challenging for the gentrification arc that is intertwined with the history of the organizations), and in terms of reducing perceived threats to the body politic relating to criminalization (especially around drugs) and costs of poverty and unemployment. Here, the organizations are at the forefront of battles to both contain and provide for young people. The evisceration of industrial employment, the decline in managed apprenticeships, and the increase in precarious employment, especially in the service sector (Standing, 2016), have all contributed to a situation in which life prospects for young people from marginalized communities seem increasingly bleak. Coupled with an increase in forms of policing and surveillance along with the criminalization of poor communities, youth from these neighborhoods often face a continuous uphill struggle (DeLuca et al., 2016). The ability of the organizations to provide for and contain these challenges means that their growth and "success" must be seen in concert with the social conditions that have produced the need for such support and care.

The term *neoliberalism* is now used as a catch-all for all kinds of economic and social restructuring, and it will infuse our analysis in the pages that follow. Here, we note how significant social restructuring (i.e., how organizations and institutions now work with the regulatory state, new psychosocial understandings of personal responsibility and self-governance, physical and economic changes to the inner city, and changing opportunities and the management of threats posed by those changes for youth) are all intertwined with the growth, need for, success, and, of course, failures of these changing YouthSites.

Education

Although the phrase "non-formal learning sector," which has certainly come into prominence in London during the past 20 years, emphasizes these organizations' place as part of a broader educational ecology, paradoxically this may not be how many organizations and actors would have defined their genesis. In both Canada and the United Kingdom, education is by far one of the largest, most established, and best resourced state sectors—comparable to health or the police, for example. Certainly, it is the major institutional frame through which our societies think about young people. In 2004, for example, when the STEP report was published, the Ministry of Education's expenditure was 13 or 14 times that of the arts (Burns Owens Partnership & Stanley, 2004).

Indeed, it was precisely the marketization of education that allowed for the growth of other kinds of educational institutions given the uncoupling of accreditation (one of the traditional purposes of schools) from institutional control. The STEP initiative was a strategic gambit to bring the activity of the organizations into the orbit of formal educational provision, thus raising the specter of their eligibility to compete for the larger pot of resources. From this perspective, we need to view the growth and transformations of organizations since 1990 in the context of the marketization of education and the way that broader trends in attitudes toward schooling, accreditation, and learning have shifted.

Although there are clear trends in the way that education systems have been reimagined and repurposed across the countries of the Global North during the past 30 years, the specific histories of Canada and the United Kingdom are very different. The authority of provincial governments in relation to the federal mandate in Canada is significantly different from the balance of local and central government in England (because we are considering London, we do not take into account regional differences throughout the United Kingdom). Questions of democratic accountability—which, on the whole, translate into questions about funding and funding allocations—are, of course, separate from questions about institutional autonomy and governance (how schools or other colleges are held accountable and managed) and arrangements for curriculum, testing, and the recruitment and training of the education workforce. In some respects, as other scholars have noted, trends throughout the United Kingdom and, for example, the province of Ontario tell very different stories over this period (Hargreaves & Fullan, 2012; see also Chapters 7 and 9 of this book).

In very broad terms, attitudes toward education within both countries have shifted in response to the declining opportunities for youth as a result of global economic changes (P. Brown et al., 2011). Both countries have seen a slight increase in the school leaving age and a decline in the values of education when measured as a form of return on investment (Goldin & Katz, 2008). The growth of precarious labor (Standing, 2016) has created a situation in which the value of accreditation has decreased as competition for secure employment has worsened. Responses to these changes in global conditions have, in both countries, focused on the management and funding of schooling and the introduction of forms of market "discipline" to improve standards through competition. In this respect, the education sector exemplifies absolutely the broader trends in neoliberal governance described earlier. Funding has been top-sliced from the ways that institutions had been conventionally supported to focus on outcome measures (examination performance or successful first steps into employment) or even targeting defined social groupings (those who had been excluded from school, those with special educational needs, those from Indigenous and minority ethnic groups, etc.). These have often been delivered in concert with area-based initiatives directed from more centralized authorities. Here, local (citywide) forms of scrutiny and control often imagined and defined what counts as education in these contexts.

Education governance over the period has thus seen a growth in forms of education institution and a dispersal of teaching and learning across franchised and other kinds of provision in an attempt to create a form of market control through regulation of outcomes. The role of community and further education colleges targeting the older student still required to attend formal education and, indeed, access provision by higher education reaching "downwards" to young people who may have left school but are not as yet qualified to go to university has also been crucial here. Because state education spending tends to focus on statutory provision, the further education and community college sector is far more fragmented, varied by region, and susceptible to shifts in labor market needs often at the local level. Because the organizations discussed in this book have tended to work with young people—broadly speaking, between ages 14 and 25 years (as noted in later discussions throughout the book, this age definition is highly varied by sector across the two countries, so this is simply a marker)—that age range means the end of both statutory school provision as much as it covers further and higher education and, most important, the focus of attention to young people who, over the period, became described as NEET (not in education, employment, or training). Attention to youth unemployment during the period and the targeting of groups of young people in the city who were defined as being at risk or in need galvanized new kinds of educational response—managing these young people at an everyday level as well as discharging broader forms of social responsibility to ensure that they could be incorporated into more positive long-term social trajectories. Nevertheless, as we will show, the transition from schooling to beyond is remarkably "fuzzy" in institutional terms (Furlong & Cartmel, 2006), even though the broader bureaucratic structure of educational provision across both countries attempts to offer services, support, and purpose for those in this age range.

The preceding discussion about changes in education has largely focused on instrumental ends—a key feature of discourse about education over the period (Ladwig, 2010)—but although this discourse frames questions of funding and organizational delivery, we also need to acknowledge changing features in curriculum and pedagogy, especially as they relate to debates about creativity, the arts, and cultural and creative expressions. Whereas curriculum studies during the past 30 years has seen a consolidation and retrenchment away from progressive pedagogy and inter-/transdisciplinarity toward more traditional definitions of subject expertise, especially in literacy studies, and a focus on core math and science knowledge, the cultural field has been utterly transformed through the growth and development of digital technologies. Although, to a great extent, such transformations have not found equivalent change in the school curriculum (Selwyn, 2010), there is no doubt that at college and higher education levels we have witnessed a growth in new forms of creative technology and communication expertise and disciplinary fields. Such changes have not exclusively been brought about by the education sector (as we discuss below); shifts in forms of youth culture and, indeed, the adaption and take-up of digital technologies in young people's lives are also driving such change, but the field of education now encompasses creative technology practices (e.g., through music technology) in ways that were unimaginable 30 years ago.

There is a whole new curriculum about the ways that digital media and the forms of cultural expression, video, music, digital arts, and work can be developed and taken to market in the hinterland of music scenes and youth culture (Bennett, 2017; Idriss, 2017), which has been advanced in the organizations as forms of cutting-edge curriculum innovation (Sefton-Green, 2013). The fields of activity we witnessed, which these organizations have sustained over time, may be incorporated into the educationalization (S. Davies & Mehta, 2013) of everyday life and play their part in the pedagogicization of cultural spheres (Sefton-Green & Erstad, 2018), but they are also examples of curriculum reform, development, and pedagogy in creative arts subjects. Formal curriculum is necessarily slightly behind any change curve, but our organizations exemplify an intermediary space between market innovation, curriculum reform, and the development of disciplinary fields as new modes of cultural expression, technology use, and artistic expression have found their place in the academy over the period of our study.

The Arts, Cultural Industries, Creative Technology, and the Creative Economy

In many cases, the YouthSites in this book had their political and social roots in the community arts movement of the 1960s and 1970s (Crehan, 2011). Institutionally, community arts exemplify both radical failure (Landry et al., 1985) and the seeds of future neoliberal transformations (Turner, 2008). The relationship between forms of collective governance, revenue dependency on state funds, the competing pressures of gentrification, and individualized consumption all meant that some of the ideological roots in community arts organizations and practices significantly reformed during the 1980s and early 1990s (Garnham, 1987; Matarasso, 1996). These are only part of the community arts inheritance for our story.

Perhaps more explicitly for many of the key actors involved, it was the art forms themselves that drove activity. This includes the ideology of community art with its belief in collective neighborhood-based expression, an emphasis on access, and cultural expression in forms and in ways, and for people who had been traditionally excluded from high art.

As we will show, the organizations promoted and, in many cases, were islands of extraordinary expertise in a range of arts. Each art form offered a particular kind of vernacular inflection. So, dance included ballet, tap, and jazz, but also street dance and dance from the African diaspora; music might involve teaching instruments, but it was equally likely to include African drumming, hip-hop, garage, and grime; visual arts might involve work with oil or pastels, but it was just as likely to involve murals; and so forth. The interrelationship between forms of high culture and popular culture, and in particular, the commodification of forms of street art and practices initially developed by socially marginalized groups, which, in many cases, drove art markets over the period, provides a key context for the kind of engagement, expertise, professional practitioners, and, indeed, forms of subcultural expression that animated the people who ran many of the organizations and drove the young people who participated in the activities. The gritty documentary aesthetic of Regent Park Focus absolutely typifies the cutting-edge of an alliance between rapidly changing technological opportunity, youth-led aesthetic innovation, and new forms of circulation and reception of media.

Key since 1990 has, of course, been the growth and domination of the internet and other kinds of digital communication and expression. In many ways, much aesthetic and arts practice found in the organizations is both a product of and a response to some of these changes at a number of levels. First, creative uses of technology have been a key pedagogical strategy to inculcate a wider set of digital literacy skills and capabilities, with arguments that digital literacy entails working across traditionally discrete modes (image, film, sound, and text; see Rowsell, 2012). This "educational" concern is deeply interconnected with an interest in supporting young people to participate fully in the wider cultural dimensions of digital citizenship through the production of all sorts of different media for social, leisure, and civic action (Jenkins et al., 2016). Bringing people together to produce forms of collective expression that can be circulated and enjoyed by peers and the immediate community harks back to some of the older aspirations of community arts as much as it looks forward to a positive vision of digital and cultural engagement in contemporary cities.

Second, the past 30 years have also seen policy interest in what has been variously termed the "creative economy" and/or the "creative and cultural industries" (Hesmondhalgh, 2012). Broadly speaking, one of the several transformative effects brought about by digital technologies has been a renewed interest in forms of intellectual property and exploitation of "the knowledge economy." Part of the refocusing of economic growth through this lens has drawn attention to the extraordinary way in which "the arts" (as they were traditionally known) have morphed into various industries under the banner of "creative and cultural industries." These have now been positioned as part of the creative economy (Florida, 2002; Howkins, 2002). Certainly, in the late 1990s and in the first decade of this century, economic policy on both sides of the Atlantic Ocean was focused on developing and exploiting talent and industry subsectors (e.g., film, television, and the games industry) as part of a broader strategy to support economic growth. The 2004 STEP report essentially drew its legitimacy from this frame: that developing creative talent across London was an important strategy to promote economic growth (Burns Owens Partnership & Stanley, 2004).

This context has also been incredibly important for the organizations. On one level, they have been seen as innovation centers, supporting cutting-edge changing aesthetic practice that could be incorporated into the broader economic agenda. For example, in the United Kingdom, the older community arts organization known as "Community Music" fostered and supported the growth of the "Asian Dub Foundation"—not just a successful band but also a way of catalyzing the voice of a whole section of London's South Asian community (Sefton-Green, 2008). Here, social policy (creating new opportunities for marginalized youth) intersected with educational strategy (developing skills in new forms of communication) and creative economic growth (monetizing talent), and so the organizations that may have had their roots in non-commodified forms of culture can then be exploited for economic ends. Values of self-expression and community empowerment thus became incorporated into the larger economic agenda of focusing talent and cultural expression into business opportunities.

Similarly, the period also witnessed struggle and debate about the diversification of creative talent (Saha, 2017). Questions about color-blind casting—the consolidation of middle-class White privileged backgrounds in many creative occupations (especially theater and music)—came into the open as questions of social justice and equality of opportunity. The new tech industry occupations began to reflect the diversity of both countries' workforces, and although the arts in particular claim a special case in terms of debates about visible representativeness, actual initiatives and programs to support progression into employment from diverse communities were frequently found in the funding behind many of the organizations' work during the period. The commitment to community and equality of opportunity that animated so many of the organizations' work with those from low-income neighborhoods merged with these wider social discussions.

There are, then, a series of art form–specific and aesthetic considerations, broader questions about cultural expression and social justice, along with changes in perceptions about economic value, growth, and opportunity, all of which came to the fore in specific policy initiatives in both Canada and the United Kingdom, particularly in the early years of the 21st century. Although policy typically in these areas would relate more to higher education or training conservatories, the ways that cultural and creative industries played a part in helping frame the terms of public discussion all meant that renewed attention was paid to the kinds of intermediary structures, systems, and organizations that were most fully articulated by the YouthSites in this book. Thus, although many of these organizations' histories lie in non- and even anti-economic instrumentalization in the community arts movement of the 1970s, by 2015, the organizations had become far more articulate and self-aware about how their presence and credibility with urban youth meant that they were in a good position to push forward other kinds of agendas. The digitalization of communication and the role of the digital in all forms of creative production and expression gave the organizations' work with youth additional urgency and educational reach.

Youth Services in the City

Interest in youth culture from a creative industries perspective brings us to the final framing context for our YouthSites: leisure and social services for youth. Mainly a feature of post–World War II social provision, and certainly galvanized by the emerging anxiety about forms of spectacular, seemingly anti-establishment, forms of youth culture on the streets in cities throughout the Global North (Griffin, 1993), funded after-school and out-of-school activities for youth became a recognized, if unequally distributed, feature of community in both Canada and the United Kingdom (B. Davies, 1999a). Although broadly a kind of welfare provision, youth services derive from a more community capacity-building spirit than simply the redress of inequality of provision, as might be more common in the United States (McLaughlin et al., 1994, 2009). In both Canada and the United Kingdom, the growth of youth services can be directly attributed to the rise of forms of youth culture in the 1950s and concern about alienation in urban environments fostered by public anxiety over post-war immigration by people of color, bound up in a series of what became known as "moral panics"—highly visible moments of civil unrest and disturbance involving young people (Dillabough & Kennelly, 2010).

Youth services were often developed at neighborhood, community, and local authority levels providing semistructured (but at that time, non-school-like) projects and activities to engage young people in purposeful collective activity. Many of these projects involved sporting and leisure facilities, and they often included the idea of a custom-designed space for young people (in opposition to the street) to allow social gathering around food. Similarly, many urban projects often involved access to nature as well as providing trips out of the city.

Key to many of these projects was a concern with harmonizing social relationships, especially between what was seen to be forms of social conflict such as between minority ethnic youth and their White peers. Building on forms of social pedagogy and drawing on principles of intercultural understanding and informal education (in this context, referring to forms of social personal and identity work; see Jeffs & Smith, 1987, 2005; Mills & Kraftl, 2014), youth services frequently developed ways for young people to come together that were marked out as deliberately differently from their formal education. With an explicit emphasis on building social cohesion, of supporting young people's transition through schooling, frequently difficult personal circumstances, and transition to employment, the youth work or youth services sector built expertise, professional training, and forms of practice. These were often funded to a great extent by local authorities, and they frequently took place in a range of voluntary and state-supported institutions, sometimes with purpose-built youth clubs, but more often in church halls or after-school premises.

Youth club practice was especially important in driving provision for young people who were deemed to be at risk, who were oppressed, or who were socially marginalized. Thus, in Canada, structured opportunities for young people from First Nations or Indigenous backgrounds and, equally, young women and also young people who identified as gay or lesbian, transgender, or queer (LGBTQ2S+) all became the focus of funded interventions to provide protective and caring environments as much to support these young people as to build solidarity through collective social experience. Frequently, the bringing together of young people for social purposes was structured around creative practice, such as making videos about "coming out" or artwork around living in minority ethnic communities in various parts of the city (Jenson & de Castell, 2010).

Funding for youth services shows a clear relationship to public anxieties around young people, with youth clubs and youth service provision of this nature being offered as forms of intervention and/or remediation. Thus, for example, the tragic murder of Reena Virk, a South Asian girl, in 1997 in British Columbia initiated responses around both girl-on-girl violence and racist attack (Batacharya, 2000; Jiwani, 2006). In London, there was concern about the growth of gang violence particularly on some housing estates.

We do not want to sound too cynical, but any quick historical overview reveals a repeated sequence of moral panics and the social response veering between public outrage and investment in poorer communities. Our organizations played a key part in this cycle of containment and intervention. Health and policing, two significant welfare sectors, thus come into the organizations' funding ecology. Anxiety around mental health, exclusion through self-identifying sexuality, gendered violence, risk of crime, vulnerability to drugs, and being recruited into gangs are all picked up by services after the fact, as it were. In this context,

YouthSites offered the state forms of intervention that could seek to work prior to any damage being inflicted.

Yet, at the same time as large, well-funded public sectors might be contributing to programs and activities to support or intervene in the lives of young people, the retrenchment of the welfare state in both Canada and the United Kingdom from the early 1990s to the late 2010s saw a significant reduction in youth services at a local level. Instead, organizations such as the ones we describe ended up becoming the new front line in social services. Whereas secure revenue funding at the local authority level might go into buildings, staff, and outreach work with young people deemed to be vulnerable in poorer communities, now the focus shifted toward the entrepreneurial acumen of the leaders in the organizations as they sought to expand services that were being closed as quickly and as urgently as demand for them increased around the three cities.

The "youth club" and youth services frame their own distinctive forms of social pedagogy and a focus on the collective social life of young people themselves to our organizations. Attention to severe social and economic disadvantage, the growth of urban violence and the controlling effects of poverty, and the criminalization of minority ethnic groups in cities have all contributed to both a need for and a realization of the value of YouthSites.

Outline of the Research in This Book

The organizations we describe and the sector that they, collectively, represent offer an original and slightly unusual lens to investigate significant changes in education, the arts, the creative economy, and youth in cities throughout the Global North. Because our methodology focuses on how the organizations themselves were institutionalized and how they incorporated older and changing forms of practice, theory, and tradition, they offer a remarkable insight into some of the most important social and political challenges to growing up today. Our historical and comparative perspective is ambitious and unusual. It has been difficult enough to find documented single accounts of community arts giving details about one organization let alone the whole culture in a particular city. Examining change in pedagogy and curriculum is difficult enough, let alone thinking of an arc from 1990 to the current day. Nevertheless, we offer this book in the belief that the depth and range of practice that can be brought into dialogue through examining change over time and across countries represent a good way to challenge scholarly debate and to bring together the very wide range of interests and fields that are frequently kept separate in academic study. Both Canada and the United Kingdom represent different kinds of welfare societies, just as the city governments of London, Toronto, and Vancouver represent different models of local authority investment and control. This, too, adds another comparative perspective to our analysis.

Building a detailed picture about organizations that have typically not necessarily been required to keep good records, and that have had to struggle to make ends meet in precarious funding challenges, involved a complex and painstaking research process. Section 1 of the book recounts in detail how we went about finding the organizations in the three cities, what patterns emerged about the ways that they came into being, how they work, how they recruit young people, how they are funded, and how they have grown and continue to survive. This section also includes an account of the ways that the organizations work as a sector and what it means to think about such aggregate activity as a field of practice. There are comparative data describing the organizations' financial returns, their rhetorical appeal, the relationship to buildings and other capital and resourcing issues, as well as a more detailed history of the story of these organizations' growth and persistence in the three cities. We chose these three cities because, to us, they represented different developmental trajectories in urban growth, from the older and more established cobblestones of London to the brash new glass and steel of Vancouver. The Appendix offers, in simplified form, a chart describing 60 organizations we contacted in the first instance, offering a synoptic overview of their form, history, and function.

Section 2 includes a series of more detailed investigations analyzing between two and five organizations in depth in each chapter, taking as the topic of each the kinds of themes, series, and politics that animated this introductory chapter.

We are aware that our topic sprawls across two continents and over a large period of time, but the practices we studied and the organizations, people, and places we visited during our research draw connections across a huge range of social, educational, political, and urban fields. This is a challenging story for us to bring together in one book. We are also aware that the histories we encountered, the leaders we met, the practitioners we interviewed, and the young people who sat down with us and took pleasure in these extraordinary places gave us a privileged insight into forms of learning, being, caring, and coping in the modern city. We learned that our YouthSites offer important and interesting insights into progressive ways of building community, sociality, economic productivity, and creativity for young people who so frequently are ignored, marginalized, and cast aside. As we write this book, at a time when belief in social institutions is perhaps at an all-time low throughout countries of the Global North, it was truly inspiring to hear about bringing young people together in such productive collective social institutions. We hope that our story will affirm a belief in the power of such action.

SECTION 1

Defining and Describing
YouthSites

The three chapters in this section offer an overview of the scope, range, and reach of the organizations that comprise what we argue should be thought of as a sector or field in the three cities of London, Toronto, and Vancouver. We begin in Chapter 2 with an explanation of quite literally how we went about imagining, finding, and excavating these organizations over a period of time since the 1990s to compare and contrast them as a data set. In Chapter 3, we offer a synoptic overview of the organizations as a city-by-city story, and in Chapter 4 we attempt to change perspective. Rather than viewing the organizations from a top-down scholarly gaze, we offer explanations from young people's points of view about why they might be interested in attending these organizations, what participation might mean for them—in general, to give some sense of what the point of the experience might be from viewpoints other than those of the funders, leaders, and policymakers.

Because we deal in the book with a large number of organizations with perhaps strange names and describe a huge amount of varied data from finance (turnover, funding, and staffing), location and building, quality and quantity of program delivery, art form specialism, public profile and reputation, educational curriculum and pedagogy, physical and welfare supports and services, and so on, we have provided an overview Appendix charting all of the organizations against these criteria. Readers may find it helpful to use this as an aide memoir as we compare organizational form and activity in our discussion of the salient themes.

Comparisons of Scale and Structure over Time and Between Countries

Our historical and comparative perspective is ambitious and unusual. It proved difficult enough to find documented single accounts of community arts—a customarily transient and document-free space—giving details about one organization let alone the whole culture in a particular city. Building a detailed picture about organizations that have typically not necessarily been required to keep good records and that have had to struggle to make ends meet in precarious funding circumstances involved a complex and painstaking research process. This challenge was exacerbated by the fact that we wanted to compare organizations not only across the cities but also over time from 1990 to the current day.

We chose the three cities of London, Toronto, and Vancouver because to us, they represented different developmental trajectories in urban growth. They have also experienced the pace and intensity of social and economic reform differently during the past 30 years. As explained in Chapter 3, different national and, in the case of Canada, provincial governments further inflected policies in education, the arts, and youth. We were trying to compare different places with their own post-colonial and community-based traditions and concerns at the same time as those places themselves were playing differential roles within national and international economic reform. Local contextual forces clearly had very particular impacts, whether they were at the level of curriculum change or policies for Indigenous youth or the place of each city within larger cultural markets.

Chapters 2 and 3—which discuss our methods and the excavation of the organizations within the social and economic history of each city and provide an overview of the aggregate role of the organizations within the cultural and educational "political economy" of each city—rest on the heuristic value of historical contrast and comparison. Although we needed rough dates to construct a form of periodicity within the very broad timescale attributed to neoliberalism—usually taken as beginning with the effects of Reaganomics and Thatcherism in the 1980s (S. Hall et al., 2013; D. Harvey, 2007)—as we explain in Chapter 3, provincial and national reform did not march together in perfect lockstep. Indeed, in all our thematic discussions—especially in Section 2—we needed to root our study in the forms of counterculture and community resistance that took root in the 1970s (Landry et al., 1985). The processes of neoliberal reform outlined in Chapter 1 are, of course, not uniform and have cumulative effects, and this, too, made a difference to the stories of our organizations and their work that they were enabled to do over the period.

At one level, we offer an intra-organizational study of institutional growth and reform that follows very basic principles of incorporation and scale. By following an organization over 30 years, we were able to see how growth and success put pressure on its internal infrastructure at the same time as comparing organizations in the region allowed us to look not just at common labor markets (especially in relationship to key staff) but also at the kind of routes that young people could follow from school through out-of-school experiences and then on to further or higher education or employment—not only in terms of linear educational or cultural experiences but also as frequently circuitous or iterative experiences within what we think of as an ecology of youth provision. Elsa Davidson's (2011) study of contrasting educational opportunities within Silicon Valley pointed to the way to understanding these organizations within an overall political economy of provision, aspiration, supply, and demand.

The idea of an ecology stresses mutual reliance on interdependent systems (Floridi, 2014). Although an organizational focus might emphasize internal coherence and progression, Chapter 4 shows how young people's perspectives on the experiences and opportunities they found and took advantage of at these places really had meaning in the context of life-wide (across moments in time) and lifelong trajectories (Erstad et al., 2016). Exploring the meaning of YouthSites in terms of these larger patterns of significance over the life course is beyond the scope of this book. However, just as forms of comparison and contrast between organizations, across cities, and over time offer a theoretical perspective to analyze the meaning of these institutions, so conceptualizing their offer within the terms of an ecology helps us understand their wider social significance.

A Field of Study

The chapters in this section include an account of the ways that the organizations comprise a sector and what it means to think about such aggregate activity as a field of practice. Chapters 2 and 3 include comparative data describing the organizations' financial returns, their rhetorical appeal, the relationship to buildings and other capital and resourcing issues, as well as a more detailed history of the story of these organizations' growth and persistence in the three cities. To some extent, constructing these organizations as analytic phenomena draws on preexisting frames about their place and purpose in different body politics.

In North America, YouthSites are regularly thought of as part of a larger nonprofit sector, albeit that term is not as embedded in the United Kingdom. Similarly, youth arts organizations can also be linked to the rise of the social economy and the third sector. The former concept is commonly used in Europe to describe organizations animated by notions of reciprocity in the pursuit of common social and economic goals. The latter nomination emerged in the 1970s in the United Kingdom and Europe to describe a developing space of collaboration between private sector groups and organizations directly or indirectly linked to the state (Nyssens & Defourny, 2013). As an intermediary space of social provision, the third sector is closely tied to the marketization of social support and the integration of private enterprise and entrepreneurial verve with the work of social and cultural provision. YouthSites grew out of a range of influences and movements, and as organizations began to form consistently in the 1970s, they would coalesce into a sector across cities throughout the world. Canada and the United Kingdom have a related history of nonprofit organization, and as in the United States, the number of groups grew in the 1960s and 1970s, often working in partnership with various branches of government to meet emerging social needs.

Chapter 2 explores in more detail the application of the term "sector" and its meaning within governmentality or administration studies. The idea of a "field" is more theoretically abstract, encompassing keenly held beliefs about knowledge domains, academic disciplines, social practices, and hierarchies of value that order such fields in our societies (Bourdieu, 1993). The idea of a YouthSite absolutely challenges the ways that knowledge about youth and provision for them can customarily be found within the fields of education or youth studies. Indeed, we contend that the emergence of these spaces forced the development of new fields as a novel kind of "sector." This theory of fields derives from the work of Bourdieu and his contribution to understanding the ways that forms of distinction matter in contemporary modern societies, and it is almost taken for granted within critical youth studies (Threadgold, 2017). That tradition also underpins much of our approach to the study of youth in the city (see Chapter 7). Indeed, the broader principles of the demarcation of fields animate a more general interest in these organizations as a classic example of the ways that conventional social institutions recontextualize and incorporate forms of difference and opposition as they exert control through longevity.

Inevitably, our scholarship was formed through our training and experience, and as Chapter 2 explains, we had to use the discipline of historical comparison to create a working theory of a political economy of YouthSites, however much that conflicted with our own internal field boundaries, as we set about finding records of the activity and impact of these organizations across the three cities.

2

The Challenges of Researching the Non-Formal Learning Sector

Introduction

We, the authors of this book, have all been actively involved in the spaces and places of YouthSites since the early 1990s as leaders and mentors, project officers, creators, and researchers. Each of us has worked with diverse art forms and with various organizations at different times. Heather worked as a theater director, dramaturge, and public high school teacher, and she has conducted research in the arts sector since 2002. Between ages 17 and 22 years, she volunteered for (and eventually directed) a youth-led organization called the Seminar on the United Nations and International Affairs; she later sat on the its board of directors. After working as a media studies teacher in an inner-city comprehensive school in London, Julian was Head of Media Arts and Education at Weekend Arts College (WAC) Performing Arts and Media College, a center for informal training and education, where he directed a range of digital media activities for young people and coordinated training for media artists and teachers. This involved fundraising, recruiting, managing teaching staff, developing new buildings and production spaces, and working on training projects with sister projects across the sector in London. After leaving, he sat on the organization's board of directors. Stuart was Director of Education at The Cinémathèque, Western Canada's leading film institute, from 1996 to 2003, where he led the development of the Film Literacy, Sights and Sounds, and Film Study Guides programs, as well as the Summer Visions Film Institute for youth—programs that continue to operate today. He has also served on the board of directors or organizing committees of various youth art and independent media organizations, including the Access to Media Education Society, the Purple Thistle, and the Media Democracy Project Vancouver. From 2008 to 2019, he was Director or Co-Director of the latter project, which involved collaboration with various YouthSites.

YouthSites. Stuart R. Poyntz, Julian Sefton-Green, and Heather Fitzsimmons Frey, Oxford University Press.
© Oxford University Press 2023. DOI: 10.1093/oso/9780197555491.003.0002

We begin with this history not only to locate ourselves within YouthSites but also because the work of making sense of the youth arts sector is not something that is easily done from above, from the perspective of policy actors and structures of governance that stand over organizations. Rather, as we outline in this chapter, this work has inevitably arisen from our own and others' experiences on the ground.

Imagining a Sector

As suggested in Chapter 1, the sum of these organizations comprising a field or a sector may be a perception shared by stakeholders, but it is not the common language of the administrative bureaucracies of the modern state. Although there have been a few attempts to make the structures of this presumed sector visible (e.g., Burns Owens Partnership & Stanley, 2004; Sefton-Green, 2008), and researchers have tried to create bird's-eye-view representations of the work of non-formal arts organizations, such attempts have often ended up struggling with their own conceptual categories (Evans & Foord, 2008; Wise, 2002).

We thus began our work with a series of "fuzzy" definitions. Mark Bray (2009) had characterized a "shadow education system," and ideas of non-formal and informal learning had been circulating for at least 30 years (Jeffs & Smith, 2005; Werquin, 2010). "Non-formal learning activity" is a designation that arose in the United Kingdom more than 30 years ago referencing a range of learning activities (arts, sports, media, and so on) that generally take place through organizations that operate beyond the parameters of formal schooling. However, scaling up projects and practices was not straightforward. The "non-formal learning sector" is not an emic concept, generally used by those involved in it, so, in imagining our sector we had to define its boundaries and characteristics ourselves, treading a careful line between creating an artificial and overly simplistic representation and becoming lost in the complexity of observed practice. The aim of our research was to describe an "object" that we could not initially define (Marcus, 2011).

We began by analyzing policy documents and media discourses that would, we thought, point to the existence of our sector. We drew key documents from our own experience with organizations and through preliminary policy-oriented research we had either produced ourselves (Poyntz, 2018; Sefton-Green, 2008) or were aware of from studies of youth learning sites and cultures. These documents pointed to other policy documents at various levels of government, as well as associated gray literature produced by philanthropic foundations working across the areas of arts, learning, and youth culture and experience. We eventually identified more than 70 policy resources relevant to our work. Media discourses about young people in London, Toronto, and Vancouver also seemed an important starting point, given our suspicion that funding for innovative forms of youth learning and development, including youth arts organizations, follows media panics about the crises, failures, and breakdowns in youth provision and youth experience. We paid particular attention to major media stories about high-profile events, including the Yonge Street riot of 1992 and the 1995 Summer of the Gun in Toronto (see Chapter 7), the beating and murder of Reena Virk in British Columbia in 1997 by a group of teenagers, and the London riots in 2011.[1]

We experimented with a word frequency analysis of this corpus (Graham, 2001) to determine how terms such as *youth, creative and cultural production, social exclusion, training, vulnerable youth, digital creativity,* and *access* and art forms, including *music, theatre,* and *media,* were produced in these documents. We searched the frequency of use of other terms, and in this way treated the non-formal learning sector as a floating signifier that we thought would nonetheless appear throughout the policy texts, even if defined by other words. This structural orientation did not, however, prove entirely productive for a number of reasons.

First, by definition, the non-formal learning sector is not overseen by any one government or industry body that collects and centralizes data about it. The absence of any preexisting consistent data thus left us wary of the view these documents offered. We could not be sure that our selection of documents revealed the boundaries of the space we wanted to investigate or merely the most well-known groups working in this space.

Second, we were conscious of the heterogeneity of the sector across cities and over time (Evans & Foord, 2008; Hesmondhalgh & Pratt, 2005; Wise, 2002). We suspected organizations in the sector shared a common set of aims and patterns of engagement with staff and young people, but we questioned if that gave their operations or their institutional form a common shape that allowed us to define organizations within a sector. Some were stand-alone companies (limited by guarantee and/or with charitable status), whereas others were connected to exhibition or performance venues, or their activity was part of broader industry engagement. Some seemed to have their own buildings, some used those of other organizations, and some were "platformed" (i.e., hosted, where core costs could be administered by the more established host organization). Many were self-governed not-for-profit organizations, driven by charismatic individuals and funded simultaneously by multiple levels of government, different government departments, and a range of third sector trusts and foundations. Amid this complexity, we were confident that what makes these organizations a *sector* is their common existence on the boundaries between subculture, industry, and government provision for youth through the arts, education, training, and the creative industries, but mapping this space proved to be a puzzle.

In the absence of any data sources about the sector as a whole, we augmented our early structural investigation of discourses about the sector with research at the organization level. We first recorded organizations drawn from lists compiled by major funding bodies, previous research projects, and individual experts (Becko, 2012; Burns Owens Partnership & Stanley, 2004; L. Harvey et al., 2002). We then supplemented and expanded this list by working with organizations to learn about who they viewed as historical and present-day peers. We continued to worry about missing key groups and projects, and this encouraged a series of iterative processes focused on the marking out of the sector through a constant back-and-forth between organizational-level view and a more structural, policy-centered orientation. Through this back-and-forth, the work of building up the boundaries of the sector came into view. As a methodology, this process seemed especially fitting given our effort to examine the consolidation of a novel space or sector of youth provision that, in turn, has also constituted a new set of relationships between civil society, the public sector, and private life.

By describing non-formal learning activities in the language of "sector," our aim was to make a disparate set of activities visible as an urban form with consistencies across time and place (cf. Duxbury et al., 2015; Garnham, 2005; Mercer, 2006; Neelands et al., 2015). We think of these activities as making up a sector because they are shaped by systems of governance and institutionalization, state oversight, regulation, and other forms of rationalization that coordinate and frame collective forms of activity. According to the *Oxford English Dictionary*, the use of the term "sector" to designate a particular industry or activity only emerged following the publication of Aldous Huxley's (1937) *Ends and Means*. The concept of a sector seemed especially germane as we increasingly came to understand that our project was marking a general shift in the conduct of non-formal learning activity: away from primarily grassroots, movement-oriented, or religiously inspired forms of organizing to professionalized, institutionally coordinated modes of organization that include substantive forms of state and philanthropic engagement (and tactical actions with private and public sector sources, to negotiate space and resources). Organizations broadly working under these conditions, with the aim of leveraging arts and learning in the service of youth provision, constitute the core elements of the sector at the center of this book.

Mapping the Organizations over Time

We then set out to produce a "theoretical" sample of these organizations—one that included the range of organization experience possible—and in the end, determined that a sample of 60 (20 from each city) would be useful as a "sampling frame" (Baker & Edwards, 2012). We could not be absolutely sure if these 60 organizations were "representative" of all organizations in the sector. As a result, we remained open to the prospect of adding or replacing groups to allow us to explore the full range of organization experience. We produced descriptions of 60 organizations, and these comprise the basis of the Appendix to this book; occasionally we also refer to other organizations in the book that we did not study in such detail. We further examined 15 case studies—across Vancouver, Toronto, and London— focusing on their existence at three points in time: 1995, 2005, and 2015. The aim was to capture the evolution and maturation of each organization within the local and national economy in order to connect organization function with changes in social, arts, and education policy.

The choice of these dates was not arbitrary but took account of the fact that neoliberalism, globalization, and digitization all coincided with our sense of the growth and consolidation of our sector. The work of social provision for young people is an old requirement in modern societies, and it is characterized by increasing institutionalization and activity led by groups working at the margins of the state, the market, and civil society. Our aim was thus to develop a method framed loosely around the periodization of state provision for youth.

In choosing our sample list of groups, we considered organization characteristics and drew on the existing understanding of the basic characteristics of grassroots organizations. This included aims, spaces, and sources of funding (McLaughlin et al., 1994). It also seemed sensible to include a spread of small, medium, and large organizations, and both older and newer organizations. As we collected data, these categories further developed to include how organizations described the young people they worked with, how they managed access to their programs, how programs were structured, and specialized art forms (Table 2.1).

At the same time, we began to see measures that captured how organizations ranged in relation to each characteristic. Thus, we began to see a spectrum of organization aims, a way of categorizing the kinds of spaces organizations were using, the framing of different sources of funding, definitions of organization size, and, of course, the range of dates when organizations were founded. As we discovered these ranges of organization characteristics, we began to use them to define the boundaries of the sector. Our data collection process and the categories we used to select and analyze data emerged together (Glaser & Strauss, 1967; Marcus, 2011). For example, we came to distinguish between the sporadic activity of small organizations, perhaps supported by another larger organization, and small temporary projects undertaken by an elite arts organizations that we took to stand outside our emerging definition of the sector.

The research began first in London. The sector categories and ranges in our data points were initially produced there and then developed to describe the sometimes different experiences of organizations in Vancouver and Toronto. This process was far from linear. The categories suited to describe one organization were not necessarily suited to the description of others. For example, indigeneity is an important issue for Canadian organizations but not for those in London. Despite struggling with our categories, lines of analysis nonetheless began to emerge. We found that although it was not possible to describe the young people the sector works with in any simple way, it was possible to describe the common ways young people were described (see below). The sector itself struggles with its self-representation—it must answer to a range of funders while taking account of sectoral sub-interests and articulating the needs and interests of youth.

Moving back and forth between researching individual organizations at three points in time and analyzing the data we generated, by city and as a whole, we

TABLE 2.1

Sector Characteristics and Ranges

Founding Date
198X	198X	199X	200X

Size (Income in 2015)[a]
Small <$300,000	Medium $300,000—$999,999	Large >$1,000,000

Income Sources
Federal government	Provincial government	Municipal government	Third sector	Private

Property
Owners	Tenants	Does not work out of a single building	Works out of changing buildings

Aims
Wellbeing and fulfillment	Amelioration of social problems	Education and training	Social change	Art form development

Art Forms
Theater (acting, devising, directing), lyrics, spoken word, poetry, writing	Dance (ballet, contemporary, street dance), mime, circus, free running	Music (instrument playing, singing, DJing, recording, producing), event planning	Film, photography, broadcast media	Visual arts, craft, design (animation, graphic design, product design)

Program Structures
Ongoing classes	Workshops, projects, and events	Accredited courses and qualifications	Individual mentoring and micro-grants

Access Structures
Open access	In schools and community organizations	By referral	By audition or selection

Labeling of Young People
Socioeconomic status	Social identity (especially race, indigeneity, gender)	Special needs, disability, or ill health	Relation to work, education, care, or policing services	Passion or talent for the arts

Types of Organizations
Traditional nonprofits	Social enterprises	Stand-alone companies	Platformed organizations	Extension programs

[a] In the Appendix, pounds sterling figures are given. Here the small/medium/large sizes are based on approximate conversion of sterling to Canadian dollars.

gradually decided on a set of characteristics and ranges with which to describe sector experience across 30 years and across three cities. The total quantity of 60 organizations gave us confidence that all sector organizations in these cities could be described according to these categories and ranges (see Table 2.1). Equally, we suggest that studying the experience of organizations in our sample would allow us to make generalizable claims about the experience of the sector as a whole, and we look forward to further research in this field.

Data Sources

In general, we drew on three sources of data: publicly available records, archives held by organizations, and data we generated through interviews and focus groups. In the United Kingdom, limited companies, including charities, file annual financial reports that are available online through the government website, Companies House.[2] In the cases of sector organizations, these reports are sometimes prefaced by a description of the year's activities and achievements, and these online records date back as far as the mid-1990s. Some small organizations, however, are exempt from having to report. In Canada, basic financial data about charities are also publicly available online through the Canada Revenue Agency.[3] The data are more standardized than in the United Kingdom but are less detailed and only date as far back as the early 2010s. Moreover, a significant minority of Canadian sector organizations are not registered charities. In the United Kingdom, Arts Council England collects and makes public a broader data set. It requires all funded organizations to report on funding sources, staffing, and participants' ages and status as Black and minority, disabled, and LGBTQ2S+ (lesbian, gay, bisexual, and transgender), in addition to "socioeconomic" background. However, less than half of the London organizations in our sample received funding, and the data are only available from 2010 onwards. No equivalent data exist in Canada.

At the organization level, we were again able to draw on publicly available material, such as organizations' websites, which often contained information about aims and programs and sometimes hosted "history" pages and an archive of annual reports. As we conducted our 15 detailed case studies, we were able to access an organization's private digital and paper archives, which included documents produced for the public—such as annual reports, flyers and brochures, press cuttings, and recordings of performances—as well as documents produced for internal use—such as research, planning, and evaluation documents. There were two main hurdles to accessing these data, however. First was the question of whether the data had been preserved. Archives were best kept in organizations that had operated in the same building for a long period and had an undisturbed space for them, and also where there had been consistent interest in documenting the activity of the organization. In these cases, the archives were a rich source of data, closely documenting the history of activities and programs. The second hurdle involved being granted access to archives that did exist. Self-presentation is hugely important for organizations reliant on donations and on public and third sector funding that has to be frequently renewed, and many organizations were understandably cautious about sharing.

When we came to conduct the case studies, in London we made visits to events and programs and conducted interviews with program directors, leaders, staff, and students. We were also sometimes able to arrange "reunion" events, including with staff from Paddington Arts and the Supporting Talent to Enterprise Programme, at which a mix of current and past staff and students discussed their history. We also interviewed key founders and leaders from WAC Arts, Ovalhouse Theatre, and Bigga Fish. In Toronto, we visited Oasis Skateboard Factory, Urban Arts, Scarborough Arts, and SKETCH, including workshops and drop-in sessions, and we attended events that showcased participant work at Urban Arts, The Artists Mentoring Youth (AMY) Project, Oasis Skateboard Factory, RISE Edutainment, Unity Charity, and Children's Peace Theatre. We interviewed facilitators and founders at Talk to Youth Lately, SKETCH, Scarborough Arts, RISE Edutainment, Urban Arts, Oasis Skateboard Factory, Unity Charity, CUE, and The AMY Project, and we did focus groups with current and past participants of Oasis and The AMY Project. At The AMY Project, we attended just over one-third of the auditions, mentor preparation meetings, rehearsals, and performances for one performance creation and production project (over the course of approximately 6 months). We also interviewed people we describe as "pioneers" in the sector, including Rita Davies, Adonis Huggins, and Loree Lawrence. In Vancouver, we spent time conducting interviews one-on-one with long-time and more recent staff, including people who had "grown up" with groups as participants, then as mentors, and later as instructors. We took part in multiday and weeklong programs and sat in on leadership team meetings with groups, including Miscellaneous Productions, as well as festival and workshop-based programs with Reel-to-Reel Film Festival for Youth. We attended a Vancouver-based Reel Youth workshop event that took place in Brampton, Ontario, and were able to arrange a reunion of sector leaders and "pioneers" who have worked in youth arts in the city and local region for significant stretches during the past 30 years.

These interview data, although they sometimes lacked historical precision, were essential to the research. The non-formal nature of the sector meant that founders and leaders were often uniquely able to tell the story of their organizations and of the sector more generally, and in cases in which there were little data available in any other form, their accounts were the only details about the organization's history. These afforded depth of understanding and offered us entry into the worlds created by YouthSites. Those interviewed for this study represent young people from across Black, minority ethnic, Indigenous, queer, LGBTQ2S+, activist, and more mainstream identity communities in the United Kingdom and Canada. Most came from cities but not all, especially in Canada.

We also drew on key gray literature focusing on arts and creative industry training, youth at risk, education and learning, city development, and cultural planning (the Vancouver Agreement 1991 and 2000), and Indigenous policy frameworks produced by various levels of government in Canada. We used this literature to extend our early policy analysis, to help frame and understand the structural conditions operating in our sector, including the role of states in labeling and representing young people.

During our first-stage sweep with 60 organizations, we developed city reports and organization profiles based on our emerging categories (described in Table 2.1), and we used these to focus attention in case studies on key organizations and themes. During this second case study phase, we developed what we called "lens-focused frameworks" based on the category building we did in the first phase of the project. We experimented with larger frameworks—for instance, thinking of our organizations as material, social, and symbolic infrastructures (Amin, 2014) in cities—and although we have moved away from these frameworks in this final text, they were crucial in helping us understand the various levels at which the organizations and the sector operated. Various concepts in critical race, gender, and cultural studies helped to shape our reading of the data, and where the evidence was available we used this literature to address the structures of racism and other forms of oppression within youth arts organizations and in the relations organizations and youth have with larger institutional structures.

Throughout our work, we have relied on our own experience to query the stories and imaginaries that animate the sector. We are open about the problem of validity at the center of our methodological work, and in response, we have worked with discursive evidence while recognizing that this and other evidence is shaped by the conditions in which organizations work, the nature of relationships youth and staff have with the organizations, and the structural responsibilities organizations have to mobilize a fundable future.

Reading How Organizations Represent Themselves

These considerations have weighed on our reading of the evidence and the kinds of claims we are able to make about the history and future of the sector. This is especially acute in relation to how we approach claims made by the sector about its impact on young people. Collecting evidence about the value of youth experience is a significant aspect of YouthSites' work. Unity Charity worked with Innoweave (the J. W. McConnell Foundation) to help it develop a measurable theory of change, driven by youth surveys and presented in impact reports, because although its mission stated that its activities gave young people tools and experiences that positively supported their mental health, and although Unity staff believed they saw those claims working in action, Unity did not have adequate evidence to support its claims. Other organizations, such as The AMY Project and SKETCH, used participant comments as part of their required reporting for Ontario Arts Council funding to help paint a picture of participant experience. Miscellaneous Productions, Vancouver, included beautiful production stills on its website—carefully staged and lit photographs of young people performing—giving a sense of the finished product. Organizations such as WAC Arts present images of students working on their projects and in classes, as well as happy, posed, post-event photographs. Much like a school yearbook, outward-facing photographs such as these, and the curated comments and data organizations brandish, are difficult to distinguish from marketing materials.

Even the data from focus groups and interviews with current and past participants needed to be treated with a certain amount of skepticism. We had permission to observe some classes and events in action, but the participants, previous participants, and staff with whom we had one-on-one conversations were always selected by the organization for us—it knew that these well-spoken individuals would share stories about the long-term and/or meaningful impact on their lives. Although we do not dispute that youth arts organizations can have a meaningful impact on the lives of many participants, we recognize that the work they do is not for everyone.

A second challenge to discussing youth experiences in youth arts organizations is the young people themselves as individuals: There are literally thousands of young people who participate drawn from many different backgrounds. The examples in this book, and especially in Chapter 4, only point toward a glimpse of what young people experience. When experiences seem to be shared across cities and organizations, we need to be cautious about how we treat them. Is the banality of lounging on the couch with friends as if at home less notable than the youth participant who makes connections that help them get paid work? Where we construct narratives of commonality, young people may be experiencing something unique from their point of view, possibly for the first time. Individual youth experiences complement aspects of our focus on organizations in order to consider a range of impacts and effects captured, measured, and expressed differently by different stakeholders for different audiences.

In general, rather than interpreting this complexity as a barrier, we pursued this struggle with self-representation as a key feature of ideological institutionalization in the sector. Claims for impact, value, and change always had to be interpreted within the matrix of claim and counterclaim, appeals for legitimation and funding, and the explicitly political discourse, all of which enmesh our data. In referencing ideology in this way, we note that ideology can be an all-consuming concept (Piketty, 2020) in social and cultural studies—one that, in certain instances, comes to delineate all or most forms of self-representation and knowledge production within social life. In our study, we work with a more modest notion of ideology, one that focuses attention on how struggles and negotiations over the representation of organizations and young people engage questions of power, its equitable distribution, and just use. We take up this notion at various stages of our analysis, and it infused our skepticism toward the range of evidence we were able to collect.

Conclusion

Together, the data we have assembled over time point to the consolidation of a new space for youth provision over the past three decades. This space operates on the boundaries between civil society, the public sphere, and the private sector, drawing resources, connections, and focus from each, while negotiating opportunities and creating programs for young people who are often excluded from such possibilities. We argue in the book that YouthSites are nimble and flexible organizations situated within the fissures and gaps in services created when formal organizations and systems, including schools, labor markets, and the media, fail young people (see Chapter 9). Organizations in the sector are resilient if often underrecognized; they are frequently led by dynamic, entrepreneurial spirits (see Chapter 8) who have demonstrated their mettle in keeping an organization's home and hearth together. The sector as a whole is a malleable space, one that has shifted as the terms and conditions of funding and support have changed. It nonetheless continues to operate in cities throughout the world, and it is this story that we aim to share in the remainder of this book. Chapter 3 describes in more detail the scope and range of YouthSites as situated within the recent history of London, Toronto, and Vancouver.

3
A Tale of Three Cities

This chapter aims to give an historical overview of the rise, reach, and fall of YouthSites in the cities of London, Toronto, and Vancouver. Readers may wish to use the more detailed accounts of the organizations provided in the Appendix to orientate themselves through what is necessarily a maze of arcane names, local funding initiatives, snapshots of activity, and broad thematic analyses. The national histories of youth, education, and arts provision in each country manifestly influence the organizations themselves. The political commitments within city politics, which, of course, fluctuate over the period, are equally influential. We aim to give a flavor of the particular kinds of influence that spurred growth—ranging from evangelical youth provision to investments in the creative technology workforce—and show how these were supported and were equally subject to changes in funding fashions, moral panics, political concerns, and social anxieties within the life of both the cities and their countries.

Without detailed knowledge about each organization, it is very difficult to make meaningful generalizations about the sector as a whole because making claims about impact on youth, arts, educational practice, or, indeed, social change requires the kind of evidence that our research collected. However, such evidence often only seems to exist in the form of local narratives that to the outsider can appear parochial, inward-looking, and sometimes only of interest to a neighborhood or community in the city or at a time far away. It is difficult to make the names of centers, neighborhoods, and postcodes resonate for readers who cannot pick up the urban myths and legends in the ways that Harlem or Watts, for example, but also Brixton, Soweto, or the Left Bank in Paris, can convey a weight of social and cultural capital. We make the case that the organizations in this "sector" innovated, synthesized, and remediated provision typically found elsewhere in the welfare state, but without a more detailed grasp of how that works in practice, such claims can always be contested.

What follows is our attempt to signpost organizations that exemplify major trends and patterns given the paucity of published accounts at this level of detail.

YouthSites. Stuart R. Poyntz, Julian Sefton-Green, and Heather Fitzsimmons Frey, Oxford University Press.
© Oxford University Press 2023. DOI: 10.1093/oso/9780197555491.003.0003

London Calling

BEGINNINGS: FROM COMMUNITY ARTS TO THE CREATIVE INDUSTRIES

Although the roots of youth provision lie in the evangelical mission in the city from the 19th century (B. Davies, 1999a), the so-called community arts movements saw the emergence of a distinct, funded youth arts education sector in London in the 1970s (Crehan, 2011; Kelly, 1984). Ovalhouse Theatre had existed as a youth center since the 1930s—run at first by University of Oxford philanthropists and then as part of the post-war Youth Service. In 1961, a radical youth worker arrived at Ovalhouse aiming to encourage young people "to consider the possibility of an alternative life pattern to the one imposed on them by . . . existing training formulas and the urban technological environment" (quoted in Groves, 2013). Over the next decade, Ovalhouse's work with young people became focused on the performing arts, and the organization became a key site in the development of community and experimental theater, particularly gay and lesbian and women's theater (see Chapter 6). Its tutors, supported by youth workers, often had experience both as teachers and as professional performers. By the late 1970s, a program for young people was established. This lasted for a good 30 years and was structured around ongoing weekly performing arts workshops and the development and performance of new work alongside schemes to support the transition from education to employment.

Weekend Arts College (WAC) was founded in 1978 by a teacher who had previously run a drama group at Ovalhouse. Frustrated because there were no routes for her talented and also often Black and/or working-class pupils into professional dance and theater training, she and a fellow dance teacher began to organize classes on Sundays. The classes were initially hosted by InterAction, a group running various community theater projects and community centers throughout London, often in squats lent by local councils. InterAction's charismatic and well-connected leader, Ed Berman, helped find performance and touring opportunities for work developed by WAC. In turn, WAC was able to attract tutors working at the cutting edge of their fields.

In the early 1980s, the Greater London Council (GLC) pursued an early creative arts policy, aiming not only to fund community arts but also to support efforts to transform the commercial cultural industries (Bianchini, 1987). It began to set up training and exhibition facilities with community groups, including a Black arts center in what became the Camden Roundhouse's building and a national jazz center out of which Community Music (CM) was formed. Neither center actually opened, but over the next few decades many new sector organizations can trace their roots from this policy initiative. Artec, for example, was set up through the London Borough of Islington and, between 1990 and 1999, offered digital media training to socially excluded groups while also operating as a production house, "artists lab," and "innovation center." It played a disproportionate role in the development of the embryonic digital media industry in London (Sefton-Green, 2008).

Organizations had previously been funded by a combination of Inner London Education Authority (ILEA), local government, and Arts Council England (ACE) money, but in the 1990s, the sector began to draw on new funding sources aimed at urban regeneration. The Single Regeneration Budget (SRB), introduced by the Conservative government led by John Major to address economic and social problems, and the European Social Fund (ESF), designed to support employment and social cohesion, both became important sector funders (Brine, 2002; S. Hall, 2016). Collage Arts was founded in 1985, and by the mid-1990s, it was drawing on both SRB and ESF funding and advocating for "the significant role the arts can play in local regeneration." It ran events and festivals and acquired studio space to house and incubate creative businesses, pioneering the model of a creative "hub." It also developed early vocational courses in community arts, sound engineering, and music business, aiming to help local people—and especially disadvantaged young people from minority ethnic communities—into work.

AT THE HEIGHT OF THEIR POWERS: THE POSSIBILITY AND IMPOSSIBILITY OF FORMALIZATION

With the election of the New Labour government in 1997, the idea that the creative industries were of economic and social importance and could be tied to an expansion or reallocation of opportunity became mainstream (Sefton-Green, 2008). Sector leaders consulted on government policy describing how the creative industries could serve simultaneously as a means of job creation and job-related skills learning and could play a part in developing senses of identity and community (Department for Culture, Media, and Sport, 1999). National funding for ACE increased, and a new emphasis was put on arts organizations to provide non-formal education and to support previously excluded groups to access their work.

By the mid-2000s, a sector was well established. As generations of its (often diverse) students progressed into careers in the arts and creative industries, it was able to draw on a changing pool of teacher-artists. Students also went on to found new sector organizations and to develop their own training to professionalize workers in the sector. New organizations grew with similar aims but dealing with new forms of creative practice. Bigga Fish was founded in 2001 by a 19-year-old running DJing and emceeing workshops in a youth club, who began to organize events so that his students had access to performance spaces. Bigga Fish grew quickly, employing as many as 18 staff members and running national tours each year that reached tens of thousands of young people. It supported a cluster of now well-known artists, developing Grime (a Black British genre of hip-hop) and also connecting this work with the most established arts institutions in the United Kingdom by running a program with the BBC to bring orchestras together with urban music and Grime artists at huge concerts, such as the London 2012 Festival (see Chapters 7 and 9).

In 2004, the first research on the London sector as a whole (named STEP [Supporting Talent to Enterprise Programme]) was published (Hitchins et al.,

2014). As noted in Chapter 1, STEP found more than 250 organizations operating in London. Together, they served 35,000 learners, 58% of whom were drawn from the Black minority ethnic (BME) community, 77% were local residents or residents of neighboring localities, 11% were disabled, and 5% were refugee community members (Burns Owens Partnership & Stanley, 2004). The research was commissioned by the London Development Agency (LDA) which, in exploring approaches to developing the skills and networks needed by the creative industries, had found in the sector an intermediary working between commercial industry and formal education—"missing rungs on the learning ladder" (Burns Owens Partnership & Stanley, 2004, p. 13).

By 2004, this "sector" had achieved a new status in relation to government social inclusion, cultural diversity, and creative industries policy. However, it had also become subject to new levels of bureaucratic scrutiny. The "open access" model of provision derived from "universalist" post-war youth service had been increasingly replaced by funding for programs targeted at specific groups of young people—those considered most "at risk" of unemployment, for example, or those with disabilities. Meanwhile, national funding often required regular renewal and increased reporting (see Chapter 9). The LDA research highlighted what a difficult position the sector occupied, even at its height. Its funding was fragmented and insecure: 81% of organizations had three or more funding sources (Collage Arts, in fact, had as many as 37 funding streams during this period), and 27% of organization funding was composed of one-off allocations, while a further 43% had to be renewed annually (Burns Owens Partnership & Stanley, 2004).

The sector had been an innovator of creative industry training and qualifications. CM was one of the first organizations to deliver training in commercial music making and production, and it had developed the first music technology course while working with young offenders. It piloted some of the first creative vocational qualifications (see Chapter 5) and different iterations of courses that resulted in its degree-level Creative Music Production and Business. WAC, meanwhile, developed the only degree-equivalent qualification in Professional Music Theatre that offered equal status to non-Western art forms, trying to insist that exam boards create new assessment frameworks to accredit these art forms. Delivering a curriculum controlled by larger examination authorities did not play to the sector's strength. In order to offer degree-level qualifications, organizations partnered with formal institutions sometimes found themselves in inequitable situations operating as "micro suppliers," unable to access the full funds needed for the work (Burns Owens Partnership & Stanley, 2004; Sefton-Green, 2008).

JUST GETTING ON WITH IT: SURVIVING WITHOUT FUNDING

In 2014, the authors of the 2004 STEP report revisited their research (Hitchins et al., 2014). Since the election of a Conservative London Mayor in 2008 and the Conservative coalition government in 2010, the LDA had been closed and a period of "public sector austerity" had begun. ACE's budget had been cut, and funding for work with formal education had declined. Most significantly, local government and regeneration and economic development funding, which together made up more than 40% of the sector's income in 2004, had been halved. The sector, however, was "just getting on with it." It continued to combine education with activities such as mentoring, career advice, startup business support, and the promotion of creative work, and its participants continued to live locally, to be drawn from BME communities, and to include those who were disabled and refugees (Burns Owens Partnership & Stanley 2004).

Organizations were having to rely more on charitable trusts and foundations and private donors, and on generating their own income. Organizations that owned their own buildings increasingly relied on them for revenue. Indeed, the introduction of a National Lottery in 1994 to raise money for "good causes" had made public sector capital funding available to the arts on a new scale and allowed many organizations to buy their buildings (Creigh-Tyte & Gallimore, 2000). Paddington Arts had received its first funding from the GLC in the 1980s for a project to make a film with young people. Continuing to run performing arts classes, initially in a church hall, it moved into an ILEA-owned building that it then secured funds to purchase and renovate in the late 1990s. As Paddington Arts then subsequently lost its local government and ACE funding in the mid-2010s, self-generated income from renting these premises enabled it to continue to operate. Its own, reduced, program of open access performing arts classes for the local community, particularly those brought together by Notting Hill Carnival, came to coexist in the building alongside a fee-paying community, public sector, and commercial users.

As smaller organizations found their own programs competing for space in the buildings they themselves owned, new organizations were founded on the basis that their buildings would provide revenue for their young people's programs. Roundhouse Studios is one of the largest London organizations, having run workshops for more than 3,000 young people in 2015. It opened in its current iteration in 2005 as a commercial venue with a young people's program in its refurbished basement, intending for the two to coexist symbiotically. Its income drew from a mix of ACE, third sector, and corporate giving and, most important, from the rental of its large main space for gigs and events and from its linked bar and catering and box office services. In fact, by 2018, public money made up only 8% of its income (see Chapter 9).

By 2014, the climate favored larger organizations in other ways too. The survival of the sector at this historical juncture of activist commitment, arts and creative industries innovation, and education and youth services was challenged. More prestigious organizations were more able to leverage private donations (MTM Consulting, 2016). At the same time, public sector retrenchment brought a new "commissioning model" in which payment for work, with young unemployed people, for example, was dependent on defined outputs, which favored larger, private sector corporations with the scale, financial capacity, and ability to take risks (Burns Owens Partnership & Stanley, 2004; Rees, 2014; see Chapter 9, this volume). Create Jobs emerged as a new kind of organization in this climate. Born out of local government initiatives to create cultural opportunities and work for local young people around the 2012 London Olympics, it went on to be run by A New Direction, ACE's London regional organization overseeing work with children and young people. Its work to train young unemployed people (and then help them find jobs) has been partly funded on a "payment by results" basis by Job Centre Plus (the British work welfare agency). WAC Arts, meanwhile, in the absence of other options, turned to formal education funding in order to continue its intensive work with young people who "struggle to find inspiration" at school. In 2014, it opened the first alternative provision free school that now runs alongside its non-formal program (see Chapter 5).

Toronto Youth Arts: From Community Music to Community Arts and Creative Cities

ORIGINS

As in London, organizations connected to youth arts have been a part of Toronto's infrastructure since the turn of the 20th century. Toronto's first settlement house appeared in 1910, and the University Settlement Music & Arts School followed in 1921 and remains the oldest community music school in the city. Similar programs developed at Central Neighborhood House and St. Christopher House. These programs were designed to serve "civic betterment" (Wasteneys, 1975, p. 5) and "Canadianization" (P. O'Connor, 1986, p. 4) as part of a series of social activities developed to target growing immigrant communities (University Settlement Music and Arts School Minutes, 1940). By the 1930s, between 75 and 100 students attended programs annually and demand grew as the schools made available "access to Western European art music (referred to as 'good music')" (Yerichuk, 2014, p. 136). By 1944 and 1945, however, the focus of community music schools shifted to "folk music," taught by people from distinct regions of the world to address the increasing racial and ethnic tensions in the city, which included more than 38 nationalities living in Toronto's urban center (Yerichuk, 2014).

In the post-war years, the non-formal learning associated with religious groups, worker and sports associations, and art groups (B. Davies, 1999a, 1999b; Jeffs & Smith, 1987) became increasingly secularized as concerns about wayward youth and youth culture emerged and states took a more active interest in the lives of young people (Druick, 2007; Ilcan & Basok, 2004; Sefton-Green, 2008). In Toronto, concern for youth populations throughout the 1960s and 1970s was part of a more general focus on local communities in Canada (Ilcan & Basok, 2004). As in Vancouver, the community turn in Toronto was significantly empowered by the National Film Board's Challenge for Change initiative and the new community art federal funding programs made available through Canada Council for the

Arts (CCA). Two federal youth employment schemes—Opportunities for Youth Program (1971) and the Local Initiatives Program (1971)—also helped channel new funds to community groups to support development of alternative arts and media programs and social services in Canada's growing cities (Keck, 1995).

In this context, a wave of new community arts groups emerged. Arts Etobicoke opened in 1973 to bring arts and culture to communities in west Toronto, explicitly including groups from various racial, cultural, linguistic, and socioeconomic backgrounds. Scarborough Arts, another of Toronto's six local arts service organizations (LASOs),[1] opened 5 years later and continues to offer intercultural after-school arts programs and projects that integrate photography, film, and storytelling in programs organized broadly around citizen learning. In 1983, Kensington Youth Theatre and Employment Skills (KYTES) opened in St. Stephen's Community Center, near Kensington Market, to serve street-involved youth in Toronto's city center. The program's employment focus emerged in 1988 when the Canada Jobs Strategy program offered funding for the provision of job skills training by community organizations. KYTES persevered through a funding crisis and transition in the mid-1990s, when Loree Lawrence joined as Theater Director, bringing a history of work with Augusto Boal and the popular theater movement in Canada to her work (see Chapter 6). By the late 1990s, KYTES offered 4-month-long, full-time (40 hours per week) programs twice a year for youth aged 16–24 years, making available theater training, life skills and job training, cooking classes, and social issues education (Kuppers, 2019). The program continued until 2003 when KYTES closed its doors due to lack of funding.

SKETCH, one of Toronto's most important community youth arts organizations, was born in 1990 as a multi-arts drop-in space. Founded by Phyllis Novak as part of the Evergreen Program at the Yonge Street Mission, Novak started project work offering street-involved youth a space to make art and do drama activities (see Chapter 8). By 1995, the work expanded, SKETCH was formally established as a business, and the organization moved into a new space where it expanded programming with support from Imago Arts, an arts advocacy organization that helps platform organizations in Toronto. SKETCH has now moved through three separate locations and is currently located in a 7,000-square-foot basement in the Artscape Youngplace building, a community cultural hub in Toronto's West Queen West neighborhood. SKETCH provides food and space for young artists, including formal training via drop-in programs, while platforming other organizations such as the Kapisanan Philippine Centre for Arts & Culture (2005)[2] and CUE (2008), a radical arts initiative dedicated to providing new young artists with the means to develop professional practices.

THE ROLE OF CITY AND NEIGHBORHOODS

The 1990s saw a more general change in the way Toronto utilized youth arts programming as part of wider city strategies. In 1990, the nonprofit group Regent

Park Focus Youth Media Centre (for its early history, see Chapter 1) was established in an effort to combat negative stereotypes in the Regent Park neighborhood. It has since offered radio, digital arts, photography and radio, and TV broadcasting programs for youth, along with a closed-circuit TV channel, Regent Park Television, for local area residents to counter the stigmatization of the community by the mainstream media.

The City of Toronto became directly involved in youth arts programming through Fresh Arts, a program that launched in the 1990s in direct response to the 1992 Yonge Street riot and the recommendations of a city commission on race relations (for more on this history, see Chapter 7). The Toronto Arts Council acquired JobsOntario Youth funding and used this to support Fresh Arts (1993) to offer arts and job training and resources to Asian, Indigenous, and Black youth to help them enter job markets. During the 1990s, federal, provincial, and local governments in Canada pursued related policies and actions that ultimately aided the development of a range of non-formal arts learning organizations. Federal policy actions (e.g., The Broadcasting Act 1991; the 1999 report of the Standing Committee on Canadian Heritage, "Sense of Place, a Sense of Being"; and the Status of the Artist Act 1992) explicitly encouraged the development of new audiences, including youth audiences, for culture and the arts. At provincial and local levels, related policies aimed to support urban youth or youth designated as at risk, by encouraging emotional support, protecting youth from violence, fostering skill development, and providing specialized services focused on the development of youth spaces in the city. This policy environment helped support the development of Lakeshore Arts (1993), another of Toronto's six LASOs; Art Starts in Toronto (1993), which began in the Eglinton & Oakwood neighborhood in response to youth despondency; Vibe Arts (1995); and 7th Generation Image Makers (1995), a culturally supportive Indigenous organization that continues to offer family- and child-focused arts programming and professional training (taught by Native artists, mentors, and Elders) through holistic learning rooted in Indigenous knowledge and cultures.

With the election of the Mike Harris-led Conservative government in Ontario in 1996, the so-called Common Sense Revolution led to the end of the Fresh Arts program, along with support for other youth arts groups in the city. The period between the mid-1990s and the early 2000s was, in fact, a time of deep retrenchment across arts and culture communities in Toronto, as austerity became the norm and support for the social economy withered. By the early 2000s, however, following the dot-com crisis in North America, another wave of youth arts organizations emerged, including the aforementioned Kapisanan Philippine Centre for Arts & Culture and CUE Arts Projects. The Children's Peace Theatre was established in 2001 in response to the United Nations' (1998) declaration of an "International Decade for a Culture of Peace and Non-Violence for the Children of the World 2001–2010" and to a rising tide of fear and mistrust that emerged in the wake of the September 11, 2001, terrorist attacks. Three years later, Unity Charity began developing programs focused on urban/art graffiti, the spoken word, hip-hop, break dancing, emceeing, beatboxing, and dance in various genres. More recently, Unity has offered other strands of programming, including after-school and community programs and community arts and culture programs that successfully blend a focus on hip-hop culture, mental health initiatives, and community building.

Other organizations emerged during this period, including Oasis Skateboard Factory (2007), a design and skateboard school that continues to operate out of Scadding Court Community Center in the historically low-income, immigrant-centered neighborhood between Kensington Market and Dufferin Grove in Toronto (see Chapters 5 and 6); The Artists Mentoring Youth (AMY) Project (2007); and RISE Edutatinment (2012), a hip-hop school and production house. In addition, two of Toronto's most recent LASOs, North York Arts (2014) and East End Arts (2016), came online.

PROGRAM ACTIVITY

Collectively, although the aims of these organizations remained diverse, their programming reflected a new and increasingly common focus among organizations established from the 2000s onward. Jobs training and skills development had long been a regular feature of organization programming across the Toronto youth arts sector. Yet, in the new millennium, market concerns, including issues of labor force development, partnerships with high-status brands, the development of professional networks and creative careers, and the development of partnerships with celebrities and other media figures, increasingly became a common part of how organizations developed and secured support for their work. Unity Charity certainly came to exemplify these developments, as did the Remix Project, an organization that has shaped the music scene in and around Toronto in recent years.

The early genesis of the Remix Project[3] started in 1999 when Gavin Sheppard launched Inner City Visions (ICV) as an urban music and art program for youth, using grants from the National Crime Prevention Centre and the City of Toronto. ICV's programming included open mics, turntables for public use, DJ lessons, space for breakdancers, and, later, a monthly MC battle as well as programs in business development. From the beginning, ICV also included a political and social justice mandate, helping give youth from across Toronto a voice; targeting and partnering with local and national politicians on high-profile youth issues including gun and gang violence; and representing Canada at United Nation–sponsored and other international events in Mexico, Guatemala, Costa Rica, Colombia, Brazil, and so on. In 2005, ICV became part of the Mayor's response to Toronto's Summer of the Gun (so called for a series of 33 shooting incidents in the city that year, many of which involved youth), and it was out of this moment that ICV rebranded itself as the Remix Project.

Since 2006, Remix has gone on to offer a host of programs, including scholarship transfer opportunities with Humber College and, in 2013, a Young Entrepreneur Business Incubator program. It has also had a leading role in the development of Toronto's urban music scene. International hip-hop artist (and Toronto native) Drake is a key ally, having recorded his second mixtape, *Comeback Season*, at Remix and launching the OVO Summit and Festival in partnership with the organization. Remix has been a regular partner with Canada's MuchMusic and with Universal Music Canada, with its own record label, Honest Music, and a radio partnership with Flow 93.5 in Toronto. By 2016, it had produced a major all-women showcase for Canadian Music Week as well as a National Basketball Association (NBA) All-Star weekend edition of the OVO Summit focused on sports entertainment, as part of the NBA's signature mid-season celebration. It has come to count among its allies national figures, including former Governor General Michaëlle Jean and Canadian actor Paul Gross, and in recent years it has expanded its operations with a branch outlet in Chicago. In this way, it is an outsized example of a new model of youth arts organization: simultaneously a media company and a YouthSite, Remix's influence crosses over between the worlds of youth celebrity, creative branding and development, and provision of media arts infrastructure for urban youth communities. In this way, it exemplified the increasing marketization of our sector throughout the 2000s.

Vancouver: From Community Arts to Youth Arts as Urban Infrastructure

ORIGINS

The story of YouthSites in Vancouver is marked by a history in media production, a tradition of community arts experimentation, and the local realities of political and cultural change. Located far from historic news and information metropoles (New York, Washington, and Toronto), yet long integrated into the Hollywood film industry as a branch plant production center set north of Los Angeles, Vancouver has been a place for film and TV production and independent media experimentation since the earliest days of cinema (Leys, 2000). Vancouver's location in the Pacific Northwest has also made it an escape destination for experimental artists. Conceptual, photo-based arts have a long history in the city—a history animated by a vibrant culture of political activism, alternative journalism, and social movement advocacy (Douglas, 1991; Poyntz, 2017).

A political shift in federal policy and funding in Canada in the 1960s and 1970s first set the stage for the emergence of youth arts organizations in Vancouver. Growing social unrest from the late 1950s and flourishing resistance movements among feminists, First Nations activists, and Québec nationalists led to a new policy orientation and funding programs from the federal government, which would ultimately help ignite the sector. With increasing support for community arts and citizen participation programs throughout the 1960s, the country's largest arts funding body, CCA, created new funding programs to bring "arts to the people" (CCA, 2007, para. 5). One of the first recipients of funds was the Vancouver-based Intermedia Society, an artists' collective that brought together practitioners from across art disciplines to explore new media and examine the role of artists in sociopolitical life. The collective dissolved in 1972, but a series of organizations grew from its ashes, including Pacific Cinémathèque (now The Cinémathèque), Western Front, Satellite Video Exchange Society, VIVO Media Arts Centre, and Canadian Filmmakers Distribution West (now Moving Images Distribution)—organizations that in different ways played a prominent role in shaping youth arts in the city.

The broadly supportive environment for community arts led to the founding of Green Thumb Theatre in Vancouver in 1975 by playwrights Dennis Foon and Jane Howard Baker. It has since developed a record of original, innovative theater for young audiences, and in the late 1970s and 1980s, it became notable as the first theater company in Canada to produce work with young actors about childhood traumas (divorce, immigration, racism, alcoholic parents, etc.). In 1979, Arts Umbrella emerged as the first sustained community youth arts organization in the city. Led by the vision and business acumen of Carol Henriquez and Gloria Swartz, it began offering theater training and other programs for 2- to 19-year-olds across the multidisciplinary arts—dance, photography, digital media, music, and visual arts. Over three decades, Arts Umbrella has offered a wide range of arts training for children and youth, and is recognized as one of the most effective fundraising organizations across the community arts sector in Canada. In 1984, a small non-profit circus school, the Vancouver Children's Circus Society, also started in South Vancouver, and 24 years later it would consolidate as CircusWest to become the leading circus performance program in Western Canada.

These groups eventually became pillars of a youth arts sector in the city, but the 1980s were an otherwise challenging and sometimes difficult period. The early 1980s brought a brutal commodity recession to the province that led to significant political upheaval and economic change. Along with this tumult, the HIV/AIDS crisis hit especially hard in Vancouver, and in the face of this tragedy, a culture of activism left a mark in the city that came to shape the development of YouthSites in the 1990s.

Fueled by the HIV/AIDS crisis, incipient environmentalism, and political theater in the labor movement, a distinctive arts activism in fact emerged in Vancouver in the aftermath of the 1980s. Patti Fraser, a long-time youth arts mentor and award-winning community artist, highlights what these influences meant at the time:

> I was . . . deeply immersed in the popular theater movement in Canada. It was the 1980s. . . . I bring that up [because] . . . that movement . . . was a movement, not a sector. And what characterized it, which is quite different from the field as it has emerged in our . . . time, is that . . . the movement wasn't there to gain

access to artistic or cultural experiences for marginalized youth. The feel of it was that it was there to define a new culture, as a representation of a movement. . . . So there was actually, when I think about now and I think about then . . . I think there was a much broader shared understanding that there was a possibility for real revolutionary change. And it was grounded in the Central and South American politics, but it did really live as a generalized understanding in many, not in all of the expressions, but it was there . . . [among] the possibilities. (Interview, 2019)

The question of whether YouthSites are a sector or part of a movement, and how this shapes our understanding of organizations and their impact on the work of youth provision, will return in Chapter 10. Here, we note that the legacies of this more radical imaginary seeped into the ambitions of a new wave of youth arts organizations that emerged in the 1990s, an influence that continues to resonate to this day. For instance, the Gulf Islands Film and Television School opened in 1995 on Galiano Island, just outside Vancouver. It offered Indigenous, street-involved, in-care, or otherwise vulnerable youth the opportunity to collaborate with independent filmmakers and theater artists on work that was distributed across the province and throughout the country. In 1996, Access to Media Education Society (AMES) and The Cinémathèque introduced separate media education and digital video production programs driven by broad conceptions of youth empowerment and critical media education. Their education programs channeled older independent and experimental film traditions as well as ideas drawn from cultural studies and the work of Paulo Freire, both of which were taught in the School of Communication at Simon Fraser University, where the directors of AMES and The Cinémathèque's programs completed graduate work.

Other youth arts programs driven by related mandates, including YouthCO HIV & Hep C Society (1994), Check Your Head (1999), Miscellaneous Productions (MP, 2000), and the Purple Thistle Centre (2001), also emerged in this period. Among these groups, MP led the development of theater workshops and full stage productions with low-income and otherwise disadvantaged youth. Elaine Carol, the founding director, started the company with a group of other women as a way to bring together theater and social issues from a youth perspective. In the company's first production, The Reena Project, MP explored youth violence in the aftermath of the murder of teenager Reena Virk by a group of youth in Saanich, British Columbia. The piece established a pattern for the company of developing projects in response to news stories and media panics about young people. This pattern has continued through a series of productions exploring racism, immigration, gang violence, drug culture, and street racing.

Other organizations, less driven by notions of art for social change, arrived on the scene around the turn of the century, including ArtStarts in Schools (1996), a less radical initiative in Vancouver then the similarly named group in Toronto. ArtStarts in Schools aimed to bring artists into schools across the province through touring and workshop programs. Reel2Real International Film Festival (1998) also emerged at the end of the 1990s, offering screening programs and, later, digital animation, artist-in-residence, and other workshops in British Columbia and throughout the country for children and youth.

DECLINE AND CHANGE

The dot-com implosion and economic downturn of the early 2000s slowed growth within the sector, but by the mid-2000s a new group of organizations emerged: Kaleidoscope, founded in 2004; Peace It Together in 2004; Out in Schools' Reel Youth in 2005; South Asian Arts in 2005; the Sarah McLachlan School of Music in 2002; and Access to Music Foundation in 2005. Vancouver's Office of Cultural Affairs aided this outburst through the 2004 Olympic Youth Legacy program that fostered engagement by encouraging youth participation across cultural life (Masters & Anderson Eng, 2006, p. 3). Part of Vancouver's campaign for the 2010 Winter Olympics included the Get Out! Youth Legacy Programs (2004–2007), which were designed in consultation with young people to foster civic participation and to support the early development of arts groups and projects. Intentionally designed to be "youth friendly" and to foster civic engagement through creativity and cultural expression, the grants program reflected a tradition of participatory civic cultural policy in Vancouver (Brunet-Jailly, 2008; Murray & Hutton, 2012; Weiler & Mohan, 2009). The Get Out! grants also reflect a pattern of relatively generous municipal funding for the arts in Vancouver, which at the time, spent 25% more on recreation and culture than the Canadian average (Murray & Hutton, 2012, p. 315). The Get Out! program was ultimately short-lived and largely focused on startup and project grants that added to the pool of youth arts groups in the city, even as the policy reinforced a pattern of project-based funding across the sector. Short-term, project-specific funding has, in general, supported the development of new youth arts groups in Vancouver for two decades, but this funding model challenges the ongoing sustainability of the sector by focusing funding on new initiatives rather than the stability of ongoing programming.

From the 2010s, creative arts and community media learning had coalesced into a sector in Vancouver, as changing learning cultures, creative culture policy, and labor market needs aligned with technology change to inspire new projects in the city (Poyntz, 2008). By 2015, the youth arts sector combined a mix of institutional forms, including after-school programs, initiatives connected to art galleries, and stand-alone institutions and projects, focused on an array of learning objectives, ranging from media education and film literacy to youth violence prevention, global education and democratization, peace activism, health and risk prevention, and the promotion of youth voice. Organizations worked across art forms (dance, photography, theater, and music) and media (video, radio, web design, and blogging), producing a mix of genres, from news and documentary to narrative storytelling and experimental theater and filmmaking. Challenges including stable funding, the lure of entrepreneurialism among policymakers, excessive audit cultures, an overreliance on unpaid or underpaid labor, and the perils of gentrification threaten the sector. But YouthSites persist as a broadly public infrastructure of care and opportunity in the city.

Conclusion

This chapter has given a brief overview of the scale and range of operations in the three cities indicating where key themes are taken up in Chapters 5–9. In Chapter 2, we explained some of the difficulties involved in "excavating" or "mapping" organizations in this sector due to the methodological challenges facing even a straightforward attempt to describe and record the range and scope of activity, let alone account for organizational operations and turnover. In this chapter, among other aims, we have tried to demonstrate how national and local (or regional) policy has influenced the development and growth trajectory of YouthSites. Organizations in the sector all share a core reliance on kinds of social funding. Equally, we have seen in all three cities inherited assumptions about providing for youth as much as the lasting impact of the community arts and other progressive social movements, even as these have been translated into new kinds of organizations that sprang up from the 1980s onwards. This is especially evident in the formation of key individuals who founded and led these organizations, and we return to this theme in Chapter 8. Similar arts and cultural industries policies can also be seen across all three cities and both countries, carrying with them a host of assumptions about what young people want and need, as we discuss in Chapter 4. All three cities exemplify at different times and in different ways cutting-edge arts and aesthetic creative practices, and this aspect is developed in more detail in Chapter 6.

This chapter has focused on describing organizations from the outside, as it were. As new kinds of institutions, they may be of interest to policymakers, scholars, and students, but, of course, they were devised both for and with particular cohorts of young people in mind. It is to their experiences of belonging, participation, and engagement that we now turn.

4

Young People's Experiences of YouthSites

Introduction

In the early 2000s, if I walked into SKETCH in Toronto, I'd be in an area of town, really well-located for the punk community, like, blocks away from the squeegee corner, blocks away from the bridge [under which there were independently led festivals and concerts]. It was by the library there. So, SKETCH, it was a place that there wasn't so many rules. The rule was like you do your dishes and somebody, usually Sue, would always be like, "Sign in, sign in!" because that was like the sign in sheet. Those were essentially the two rules. Everything else was like, "make something. You need to chill out, you need to play music." So it was a space where you could, there was always the supplies to do what you wanted. And for so many youth for so many of the situations they're coming from, to just have a space to be without participating in a formal program. It was a very different space. . . . And it had really healthy food, like it was, as opposed to like mayonnaise and jam sandwiches that some places give out, with white bread . . . it was just like, healthy food, cool people, just like an open-concept space, very well-located. . . . .

At the time, SKETCH still ran a three-day-a-week open studio program and people for those afternoon workshops, there were 30 people a day, and sometimes more.

—AMELIA, former SKETCH participant

In 2017, when our team visited SKETCH at the Artscape Wychwood Barns, there was more security, and there were forms to fill out, and there was tracking. When our team first toured the studio spaces in the basement, it was not during a programming time, but a few people were working on music mixing projects, and the open and inviting kitchen included an "essentials cupboard" from which

YouthSites. Stuart R. Poyntz, Julian Sefton-Green, and Heather Fitzsimmons Frey, Oxford University Press.
© Oxford University Press 2023. DOI: 10.1093/oso/9780197555491.003.0004

participants could take as they needed. The facility included spaces for music, Photoshop/computer areas, a dance studio, a woodworking area, a paint area, a kiln and pottery room, a screen-printing area, a textiles area, a live green wall, and gender-neutral washrooms. Signs reminding people that SKETCH was a safe and inclusive environment were posted on the walls. Later, one of our youth research assistants participated in a drop-in night when approximately 40–50 young people came and went. No longer "punk," or dominantly male, she observed that there seemed to be a gender balance and that nearly all the participants appeared to be non-White. Sue, still a member of staff, gave her a tour of the space and reminded her that if she stayed, she had to create something—the same message as in the early 2000s.

> Supper included meat and vegetarian options, water, coffee, and juice. I noticed that people were heaping plates full of food and that everyone was really enjoying themselves as they sat together to eat. Once I got my plate, I joined the two guys I met as I first walked into the building. . . . Everyone was talking amongst themselves over supper and there was no rush or schedule.
> —Madison, research assistant

Our research assistant chatted with youth participants about what they had been working on (silk-screening T-shirts), and they invited her to help. They showed her how to use the equipment and also the techniques to get the best print. Eventually, our research assistant moved over to the painting section, where a facilitator was sharing watercolor techniques.

> People were interacting with each other throughout the whole session, obviously having known each other for some time or at least met a few times prior. People seemed to come to interact with other artists through the night. Some came to work on specific pieces, and some came just to socialize and enjoy the space . . . some went with a sense of direction [straight to the kiln or the screen-printing room]. Others, who had not navigated the space before, like myself, were invited to participate in art sessions and either stayed or chose another space. As the night came to a close, facilitators went around and began cleaning up any coffee mugs that might be sitting around from participants, and people started to drift out of the space and leave. Folks were told that they could leave their art (if it was still wet) and pick it up the next day if they wanted to. The space was very homey and I got some really positive vibes as the night went on. . . . The space was very open and welcoming for youth artists and seemed to be a place that people often returned to happily.
> —Madison, research assistant

The previous recollections and field notes of visits, both from SKETCH in Toronto and approximately 15 years apart, remind us that programming structures change, spaces change, and young participants change, even if the youth arts organization itself endures. Yet past participant Amelia and our youth research assistant

Madison identified similarities: There was good food, there were positive youth relationships, the young people could "hang out" in a place where they felt comfortable, and everyone was urged to "make something." Most of this book seeks to analyze the youth arts organizations themselves, but this chapter is different. None of these organizations would exist if there were no youth-driven demand for what they do. To flip the focus of inquiry from the organization to the young participants, we asked, How do youth experiences shape those organizations?

To answer that question, this chapter explores what matters to participants: Why do thousands of young people voluntarily spend their time at YouthSites, choosing to explore creative energy, hone skills, and develop relationships there, and not somewhere else? The previous two chapters explored, first, how we constituted the field of YouthSites through our research and, second, how policy, funding, and provision created organizations within the local contexts of each city driven by a mixture of top-down welfare concern as much as by community activism. Here, we explore the affective experiences and reflective responses that speak to why youth arts organizations have become an essential aspect of urban infrastructures for youth and why so many young people value their experiences at YouthSites.

There are no simple or "reliable" methods to capture youth experiences, and given that we are interested in a 30-year history, and we did not set out to research contemporary responses over time, we make two methodological caveats. First, the chapter reflects on the meaning of youth experience as defined by the organizations. We explore how they used evidence to support claims about the value youth arts organizations made in youth lives. These can be part of a rhetorical appeal to funders (as we discuss further in Chapter 9), but also highlights how the organizations themselves operated with cultural norms about who youth are and what they wanted and how they, the organizations, came to these beliefs. The reflexive construction of an ideal youth experience is thus part of our argument here. Second, we have synthesized what current and past participants told us about their experience from field notes and observations to enable us to generalize about what "youth experience" might mean collectively rather than just within individual life history narratives. We recognize our role in this filter. Numerous other researchers have prioritized youth arts engagement and outcomes (Campbell, 2019; Wallace Foundation, 2013; Wright et al., 2006), arguing the value of turning attention to how young people express the significance of youth arts organizations in their own words and through their own creative expressions—even if it is filtered by the organizations or by the capriciousness of memory and reflection. As Chapter 3 showed, we further believe that analyzing youth engagement with the specific organizations we studied is essential for a thorough understanding of these organizations and, therefore, the sector as a whole. YouthSites do not exist because of government mandates, laws about education, or city-sponsored anti-crime or health and wellness initiatives, although those may certainly influence organizations. YouthSites organizations exist because of the young people who participate in them, and so this chapter turns a spotlight on them.

Timelining Engagement Across YouthSites

We identify four stages of participation in a youth arts organization: arrival, participation, exit, and post-departure involvement or reflection. Some young people respond to active recruiting and apply; some are directed by welfare services and career counselors; some are eligible because of their "at-risk" status; some attend auditions or drop in; others participate in a school-based (no choice) activity and then choose to continue to be involved; and still others arrive with the intention of disrupting the activities, and then they choose to stay. Eldora's story about her arrival at Paddington Arts, London, is the latter. She explained,

> It was literally walking down the road being dysfunctional . . . with my two mates. . . . The church hall was open with this big sign saying "Come and do some Dance and Drama" and we actually went in there to make trouble. We were like "We've got nothing to do, let's go mess up . . . Dance and Drama, it's for wusses, who want to do that?" And we went in there with 100 percent intention to cause havoc, by any means necessary. . . . So that was our mission, and the mission kind of turned on us because we enjoyed the bloody thing! Which was a nightmare. And it was basically between the three of us who was going to admit they enjoyed this the most, or first. . . . So it was crazy that we went in, really enjoyed it, came out smiling saying "When is the next session?"

There are no dominant models of recruitment. Some young people choose to move on to other things or do not get accepted into the organization. For example, Meg Solis, a Miscellaneous Productions participant, told us,

> I went with my friend and we both got in and she didn't necessarily last that long because she didn't feel like the program was a fit for her. She had other things going for her but I felt that it was a good fit.

Once young people participate, the unfolding youth and arts organization relationship can continue in different ways. If the space is a drop-in, young people will participate as long as it suits their interests, lifestyle, and capacity to attend. If there is an application process, the activity is typically finite, and participants may move on once the activity or project is complete. There may or may not be opportunities for re-engagement if they choose, perhaps applying to another project or continuing as a youth mentor. At some point, even if the activity is ongoing, young people will age out—they may no longer be allowed to participate as youth. Here, again, some past participants found ways to participate through alumni activities or as volunteer or paid staff, as Amelia, Eldora, and Meg did.

The introduction to Section 2 that follows this chapter notes some of the literature investigating aspects of participation. There is very little overview research about the moments of recruitment or sustained participation across organizations, yet making a case for participation is often central to the organization's narrative about itself.

Counting and Representing Participation

Participation numbers might help us set a scale of youth engagement. For example, we know that when young people keep returning to participate in an organization's activities, they must value the experience. Yet, if activities are offered in and through schools (as is often the case with Reel2Real in Vancouver or Unity Charity in Toronto), young people do not participate by choice: the activity is mandatory. If activities are offered to participants as a one-time fixed-term experience, as with The Artists Mentoring Youth (AMY) Project in Toronto (participants sign up for a specific time-based program), Weekend Arts College (WAC) Arts in London (some project participation offers credentials), or in the Oasis Skateboard Factory in Toronto (a limited number of students sign up for a term or two to complete school), the attendance numbers alone cannot describe commitment to the program. Progression across separate programs within the same organization is also not captured. Furthermore, a focus on completion suggests that there may not have been value for participants who withdrew for a myriad of reasons. At drop-in spaces such as SKETCH, or spaces where multiyear participation is possible such as Paddington Arts, participation numbers do not necessarily report repeat visits from individuals or how many young people are visiting the space more than once a week. In addition, when participants "age out" of programs because of the organization's mission and funding parameters, we cannot know if past participants would have continued to find the organization meaningful beyond the limits of permitted participation. Depending on the scope of the organization's activities, and its engagement model, staff may have faces and stories to put to these numbers, but participation numbers alone do not provide much insight into questions about youth experience.

The Appendix contains such data as we were able to collect counting rough student numbers at each point in time to give some sense of the range and variety of attendance. Note that this counting performed a strategic function for the organization in terms of claims made to funders and is not detailed enough to show participation over time or depth, meaning, and quality of experience.

In addition to tracking participation numbers, organizations produce outward-facing documents, and now, websites and Instagram and other social media pages, to provide a window onto the youth experience. Although they contain information about the organization's activities and may use numbers and qualitative data to support claims, these documents generally have three purposes: to recruit more participants, to attract donations, and to positively report on activities to reassure supporters about the value of their contributions. These documents often represent youth experience in emotive terms—they show cute pictures, record young people's expressive outputs, and use imagery to portray dynamic, motivated, and engaged youth, as discussed in Chapter 3.

We therefore now examine how organization claims for their outcomes relate to how young people describe their experiences in youth arts. We then explore how care and community are fundamental to how participants discuss youth arts.

Organization Outcomes and Youth Experiences

Organizations use the evidence they have about young people's experiences to show how they address individual life skills and well-being, broader social benefits, training, community cultural change and the development of the art form, and creative production. Although this language and these categories of impact derive from the policy or welfare discourse about forms of provision and care, not bottom-up "emic" explanations for and about young people's experiences, as categories they infuse the ways that youth seek to explain the value of their participation. We thus use this framework to show the interplay between the ways the organizations tell stories about themselves and the young people's version or their part in these stories.

INDIVIDUAL LIFE SKILLS AND WELL-BEING

Individual life skills and well-being are important to funders and young people alike. Yet statements such as "As a result of our community program, 88.6% of youth strongly agreed or agreed that they had developed confidence in their own skills and abilities" (Unity Charity annual report, 2017) or even "I used to be a very shy kid . . . until I stumbled into the program. It drew out the outgoing confident, and passionate side of me that I had never felt before" (Kareen Wong, quote from Unity Charity annual report, 2017) do not offer a sense of the youth arts space and the experiences that led to those outcomes. In our conversation with Adrian (Unity, Toronto), he reminded the others in the session that

> you might run a workshop for one week, he or she or whomever comes back for the second week. There has to be a reason that this person comes back for the second week. . . . Sometimes there's so many youth in a program that it's, like, really hard to keep track of everybody. But there's a reason that this person keeps coming back week after week after week. And we just have to keep that in mind.

Something young people value happens and is available in youth arts organization spaces and programming, but what exactly is it?

Fio (at the time of writing, a current AMY Project participant) linked developing life skills and well-being directly to the opportunities she experienced while being a part of the youth arts organization. She noted that the project aimed to be barrier-free, crossing boundaries found outside within the organization's space. She described the caring and feeling cared for experience as a significant base to develop life skills and a sense of personal wellness. For example, she explained that providing her with public transit to get to the venue (which took her a full hour each way) and really good meals supported her, along with weekly check-ins: "To share how your day was or how your week was with everyone really makes you feel like you matter." She reflected on the weekly writing prompts in which participants respond in creative and artistic ways and which can then be shared. Along with gaining collaborative creative skills through writing and sharing, she acknowledged how AMY taught the young people to self-advocate and to lift others in the room:

> We made a list of how we can support each other and in ways that we need support. And so then everyone knew each other's bucket so then we can help each other that way and it really helps you develop artistic sense, but in a really safe space.

Rofiat, another 2018 AMY participant, expanded on Fio's comments: "Like, I have troubles at home. . . . AMY is just the space where I'm free from home, I'm free from school, I'm free from everything. I don't have to think about anything I just have to be in the moment."

After sharing their meal, all the AMY Project participants, facilitators, and any guests clean up and wash the dishes together. Then together they silently engage in a ritual of hands-and-knees floor washing, ensuring that everyone is involved in preparing the space anew. They sit in a full group circle, do their check-ins, and then the first hour is devoted to developing theater creation skills (e.g., dance skills or dramaturgy). The second hour is devoted to working through the creative work they produced in response to the prompts Fio mentioned, with a view to ultimately moving some of those pieces into a collectively devised performance.

Approximately 8 years after she attended The AMY Project, Amber told our research team that the creative writing and storytelling part of the work—which, of course, was an aspect of the building blocks for making a show—was also the beginning of her own wellness story, and one that carried forward beyond the project itself. She explained,

> Going through that process and telling that story, I think it started a journey of healing, I guess, and trying to unpack all of that stuff and how its impacting me. . . . It's just been a blessing and a curse but I am grateful that it happened because I don't know what my life would have been like if I had never paid attention to it or recognized it.

Past participant Fitz also commented that the personal creative development work was therapeutic, even though it was not therapy (an idea also asserted by Phyllis Novak of SKETCH; see Chapter 8). A significant aspect of the youth experience is feeling heard and learning to listen, and also learning to value their own stories and lived experiences as relevant and meaningful pieces of who they are, who they are becoming, and how they relate to community.

Sometimes youth arts organizations use a language of "empowerment" to talk about the way that youth arts experiences amplify participant voices and provide platforms for them to be seen and heard and to shape their communities. When young people feel like they can be critical and question the systemic injustices that influence their lives, the way they use their voices can be different too. Amber observed that The AMY Project approach to art-making from personal stories humanizes other people, especially because people in the program come from so many "different backgrounds and stuff like that." Furthermore, it creates "an alternative to institutionalized learning, which sucks, and is racist, and all of these things," and instead offers something she calls "anti-capitalist," "accessible," and "sustainable." Amber's experience suggests that she sees the experiences she had at AMY operating in her own life in a "sustainable" way and that she sees herself subsequently pushing out into the broader Toronto community and making changes.

When Loree Lawrence was at Kensington Youth Theatre and Employment Skills (KYTES), a Toronto theater company working with street-involved young people, she asked participants to adhere to schedules and routines similar to those expected in 9-to-5 jobs so that they would know that they could be successful in those spaces, and they could then critique them from a position of confidence. Similarly, teachers Craig and Lauren, at Oasis Skateboard Factory, discussed the importance of knowing knowing how to build networks, learning to work capitalist systems to their own benefit.

It is telling that participants emphasize the ways that the organizations build them up and support their well-being differently when they are still participants, compared to how they reflect on the value of the organization in their later lives. In her study about KYTES, Lawrence (2006) observed that although many of the youth observations lack the "transformative tone" funders are looking for, participants explain that KYTES gave them confidence, resourcefulness, and helped them embrace some goal-oriented qualities. She noted two KYTES participants' comments:

> It's taught me not to feel bad about my failures. "So what, it didn't work out, move on." It helped me in life to realize that I don't have to condemn myself to shit because I didn't do something the way it's supposed to be done.
>
> KYTES was able to show me that there are positive things about me. I can go out and do my own thing and fulfill my own prophesy instead of proving everybody back there that they're right (pp. 69).

Lawrence's research about KYTES also suggests that for some young people, the life skills and sense of well-being they gain through youth arts program participation may seem quite subtle to outsiders because they are not always sensitive to the range of different life experiences:

> KYTES had a role in my transition from being on the streets and being in that sort of world where I expected less out of life. It was easy for me to think about tomorrow. I am resourceful, that's how I describe myself now. That's quite a skill, to get up and go (pp. 70).

TRAINING

The way youth experienced the training offered by youth arts organizations was deeply bound up with a perception of relationships. These included mentoring (see Chapter 8), developing professional networks that would otherwise be inaccessible, or finding ways to connect with a professional arts community. As we describe in Chapter 5, claims that organizations made regarding the training and skills they provide young people varied significantly from site to site: Some programs offer credentials, whereas others offered particular arts-based skills or to help participants develop generic employability skills. Young people may experience leniency and/or patience with regard to out-of-program life challenges, or may be able to access resources to make regular participation easier, but the organizations offer rigorous pre-professional training, which demands commitment. Past youth participants discussed the training in ways that valued elements of training *with care*.

Meg Solis was in grade 12 at her high school when she noticed a flyer for Miscellaneous Productions that promised "you get X amount of worth, like monies worth of training but for free. And I was like, 'What's the catch?' There's always a catch." Meg was growing up in a lower income family in East Vancouver and was curious enough to attend an audition. She was suspicious, but because the poster claimed "no experience necessary" (she had never previously been able to afford to build the experience she would have needed for other auditions), she thought it was worth trying out. The economic accessibility of the training and the fact that it was not too far from where she lived helped because her parents would have forbidden her to travel to what they perceived as a more dangerous neighborhood. In fact, Miscellaneous Productions reduced as many barriers to offering training as possible so that there really was no "catch."

Similarly, when Mercedes applied to The AMY Project, the professional training aspect appealed to her. She had grown up in a low-income family in Toronto, but her mother could see how much Mercedes loved the arts and, from a young age, registered Mercedes in every free arts program she could. The AMY Project, which promised fully mounted original productions, was a step beyond what Mercedes had done before:

> At the time . . . the importance that I placed on AMY was the opportunity to, like, just get a sense of the professional world. Like, I was already accustomed to stages but the professional stage, that was, you know, that was a bit different. The idea of a stage manager and a stage sound board and an actual stage and everything . . . so just learning the ins and outs of the industry.

The possibility of high-quality learning appealed to this young woman, and the "care" aspect of training was apparent right at the beginning of the relationship between her and the organization.

Formal life skills may be necessary for successful employment in a general sense, but some participants, like Meg and Mercedes, sought high-quality training for its own sake, as well as for the way it contributed to a portfolio in contrast to conventional credentials. Phyllis Novak, Artistic Director of SKETCH, explained that as participant demographics changed, so did what they were looking for.

In the 1990s and early 2000s, the street-involved youth, often from Toronto's punk scene, were more interested in having a safe place and to discover a sense of self. However, in the early 2000s, when young people needed a place to hang out, listen to music, and "make something," Novak noticed that "it just seemed different, something was different then, I don't know what it was." She realized that few young women were taking advantage of the spaces, so SKETCH worked with a Status of Women grant in 2009 and learned that young women, especially racialized women, wanted SKETCH to help them build tangible skills that would lead to employment. Novak remembered young women were saying "I need to have something that's going to advance my opportunities" and "I need something constructive that's going to take me from A to B." With the exception of the 1990s Drug Project, which had an 8-week trajectory and demanded commitment, participation in SKETCH is "always designed with an off ramp, so it's like enter and exit as you please." Although Novak named specific young people from that era who also developed skills that they used to start businesses (in construction) or study at university (we spoke to one former participant who decided to study geography), the need to provide tangible outputs had become important. In 2011, participants wrote comments that inspired Novak: "Why can't SKETCH be my school?" and "SKETCH is my job training center." Although SKETCH does not offer credentials, the idea that it could be a space that responsively developed training opportunities to meet needs articulated by the young people themselves was perceived as a form of care.

Other programs, such as WAC's social inclusion program, were specifically set up to nurture young people who do not—and perhaps are unable to—fit into a more typically structured education program. Camille Curtis of WAC Arts (a former Paddington Arts participant herself), explained,

> The whole point of WAC Arts is to use the arts as a tool to re-engage those young people, to get them back into education, to build confidence, or to find skills that were always there but which hadn't been nurtured.

Although WAC Arts' outward-facing literature highlighted now famous performing arts professionals who had initially trained there, Camille chose to describe a boy on the autism spectrum who arrived at WAC Arts, "sliding down the corridors," and her initial response was "this is not going to work." And yet, she enthused that this young man is excellent with media, mixing unexpected combinations, and playing hip-hop on the piano:

> Every young person deserves an opportunity . . . [and] should be able to flourish whereas if you are in a mainstream environment sometimes these people are overlooked. [At WAC, with so many fewer participants than a typical college (60 instead of 1,000)] . . . you can give them specialist time, you can nurture them, you can know exactly who everyone is, you can deal with issues much faster, so everyone feels special and it feels like a family.

Meg Solis told us that after she had left Miscellaneous Productions to extend her training at Capilano College (a program she believes she could not have done without the training from Miscellaneous), the opportunity to share training with youth participants brought her back to Miscellaneous as a staff member. Initially, she was teaching dance and working as an assistant. Yet, like Camille, it was impossible for her to disentangle training from a focus on relationships and care. She explained,

> I think it really was being able to help other youth who were . . . might have been in my position that like they . . . they didn't have anywhere else to really do any of this training. But also, I felt that I had a unique . . . a unique approach to things because I could approach things from their perspective. . . . I felt that it was something that I could offer that not many other professionals could. . . . I wanted to help kids who were like me and I think that I still came from, even if I didn't have a lot, I still think I came from a privileged background because there's a lot of, you know, youth I know and don't know, who are way worse off and they . . . they don't have any privilege and they have a lot of, you know, really bad experiences. And coming to the program is one of the only stable things in their lives and it's the only place where actually people check up on them and they care about them. And a lot of the times . . . a lot of the times with a bunch of youth, we're the only ones who really care about them because they have either very tumultuous relationships in their lives or they're just not in a good situation where they have any support and we become a support system for them and a community.

Current and past participants describe their experience of training as tightly connected to the way they experience relationships of care with facilitators, networks, and the supportive community they built that lasts beyond the bounds of the program. In a focus group discussion with past AMY Project participants, Amber noted that the network she developed at AMY led to a variety of opportunities: "[You could say that] I went to art school through a bunch of community-based art projects and AMY was my first year or something." She explained that AMY helped open doors to Paprika, The Remix Project, "and a bunch of other programs all over." Her connections with the AMY network brought her back to AMY to do headshots and graphic design as a contract employee: "I think building genuine connections and building community and sustainability and sort of sharing those resources amongst all the people that come though AMY. So that it's continuously like a synergy and like a continual building a cycle."

Mercedes, who might be seen as an AMY Project success story because at the time of our conversation, and 7 years after she left AMY, she was employed full-time at the Stratford Festival, explained,

> So what I've valued and continue to value, I should say . . . is the family aspect, that I have those connections that I made, and how they've . . . they can also

translate into networking opportunities. Like, not to say that I'm, like, "no I'm only sticking around cause I may need something," you know what I mean? But you are aware that if you do need help, they will extend that.

For many youth arts organizations, mentorship and networks are an extension of the training they offer, and the young participants experienced these as opportunities to connect with people who feel like a caring family. Unlike Amber, Bessy had the opportunity to attend university theater school and also The AMY Project. Her words capture how her experience of care was simultaneously an aspect of how she experienced training:

> Both of them offer so much but the way that they go about it is just very different and, um, yeah, I feel like for theater school they don't really like check up on you until you to do something good like, "ah now we want you because now we want our future students to see that . . . you came from our program" . . . like making them look good. Whereas AMY—they just care about you, they care about people and when they want to promote somebody doing well, it's genuinely because they care.

COMMUNITY CULTURAL CHANGE AND ART FORM DEVELOPMENT

Two common claims that youth arts organizations make is that their programming contributes to cultural change in the community and to the development of novel grounded art forms (see Chapter 6 and below). Adrian, from Unity Charity, noted that those shifts are felt within spaces and among the young people who attend the programming, who support one another, and who no longer "beef at each other or steal each other's stuff."

If organizations aim to impact a city's culture, such ambitions significantly influence the character of participation. As Novak explained in 2011, the SKETCH approach begins with a respectful relationship: "We assume people are creative and that they have something to contribute." Jason Samilski, creative director at CUE, a former SKETCH participant, claims that CUE avoids tokenizing youth and embraces their creative ideas and does what it can to support them with more than words. Because much can happen in these young people's lives in a short time, CUE offers very quick turnarounds for the micro-grants it distributes in order to establish positive, action-oriented experiences. He explains that if someone has an idea to do something unusual, such as a special event,

> we can say, "Oh, someone needs a space to do what for the night? That sounds lovely. Who wants to stay late? Oh, can we, Yo, can we throw some money at this so we can get some food for them for the . . . for their event and stuff? Okay cool, let's do it." Boom, done and get back to them the same day, you know?

In other words, young people's ideas are heard, embraced, and can become reality— because of the support they get from organization staff, they can influence their space and their community in tangible ways. Perhaps most significantly, Samilski argues that the fact that youth art gets a professional-style gallery showing with an opening event, and an installer to help hang their work in their gallery, means that young people can follow the entire grant trajectory from receipt of funds through to creation and then to exhibition. Time and again, youth arts organizations provide opportunities for youth participants to see themselves in the professional art world—and the art world sees them too. Notably, Lensa Denga, of Urban Arts in Toronto, pointed out that when young people's creative contributions and talent are seen, some people in the community try to take advantage of that. They may ask young people to perform for "exposure" and "opportunities" and to make their own event look connected to youth communities. Denga and Samilski try to ensure that their youth participants are treated with respect, and, where appropriate, they advocate for participants to be paid for their work. The young people are seen as artists and contributors, and they see themselves that way too.

Uncomfortable youth experiences also take place during youth arts organization events (see Buckingham et al., 1995, Chapter 4), and some of these can be damaging to goals of community cultural change. We witnessed such an event during a Reel2Reel Festival in Vancouver, widely attended by schools. Following a film presentation, there was a facilitated discussion during which only White, male students participated in the conversation, and two students spoke out problematically. Student A invalidated the female voice in the documentary, saying that her speech was "only emotional" and not based on facts. We noticed that the students seated nearby were visibly uncomfortable. They grew agitated as Student B began to make statements undermining the idea of transgender rights, questioning what is meant by "barriers to access," and finally, when the conversation turned to Black Lives Matter, asserted that White people get shot more than Black people. Around our researcher, racialized female students took out their phones and muttered "Google it," and students shuffled and shook their heads, but Student B's voice was allowed to command the room. No one, neither the students nor the facilitators, challenged him. We imagined how silenced, marginalized, and invalidated it made many young women and racialized young people feel. Although the Festival aimed to offer opportunities for youth-driven, thoughtful, critical discussion about issues of interest to young people, in fact, the space perpetuated divisions and enabled microaggressions to go unchecked. Positive youth experiences in youth arts organizations require, among other things, expert facilitators, and an opportunity for young people to feel their experience is part of a positive impact beyond the space is far from guaranteed (Kirshner, 2015).

BROADER SOCIAL BENEFITS

Although YouthSites' primary activity may be sharing arts practices, they may also be expected to help young people finish high school, engage with healthier life practices and avoid substance abuse, give young people "somewhere to go with something to do," and discourage youth delinquency, including petty and violent crimes, while at the same time providing a safe place. RISE Edutainment founder Randell Adjei had only been running his spoken word events in Scarborough for 3 months when tragic gun violence broke out just blocks away. Some girls who had attended his event night told him that they were there because they knew it would be safe, and he realized how important this was to young people in his community. Like the girls who spoke to Adjei, some young participants reflect on how the youth arts spaces offer them alternatives, even if some may prefer not to talk about those kinds of outside pressures.

Adrian, who is now a dancer and educator on staff with Unity Charity, used to go to its drop-in space at Yorkdale as a participant. He spoke about what it was like to participate, highlighting that for him, it was great that the drop-in was available locally so that he did not have to take the bus long distances in Toronto. He also explained that unlike the parachute programs Meg Solis describes in Chapter 8, Unity commits to specific locations and brings in significant resources (e.g., quality sound equipment), "and we want to do long-term work there, or we try our best to, and the kids do see this." His experience as a youth at the drop-in space was that

> we were allowed to be what we wanted to be. We were rowdy, a wild group of kids. We would dance for, like, three-and-a-half hours non-stop and then go to another place to dance. It just provided us with a space to be, like . . . it kinda guided us to be, like, hip-hop is about respect and about hard work, resiliency, and we kinda took it in. Because without that space to guide us, we would have just been, like, no, screw this, or we would have sessioned at another spot.

Being in a space that promoted respect helped people feel safe, even if they were just there to hang out rather than to dance:

> It builds community and family in those spaces. People really get to know each other rather than have, like, issues. They would genuinely look after each other. So it changes the culture, the spaces as well. But it takes time. A lot of time.

Young people explicitly value the way that arts organizations can offer an alternative, youth-focused space that feels safe and promotes positive community values. The ethos of mutual care, combined with the convenient location and a focus on respect, kept young people coming back to dance. A youth participant told Unity, "In the smaller picture you are changing kids' lives. . . . In the bigger picture you are contributing to a happier, more peaceful society for now and the future" (quoted in Unity Charity annual report, 2017).

MAKE SOMETHING

At SKETCH, for more than 15 years, Sue has been reminding youth participants that they need to *make something*. Chapter 6 discusses the significance of feeling represented and heard, but even more than amplifying youth voices, developing brands that attract attention, and having art shows in public galleries, spaces to practice and perfect dance moves, or platforms to perform a spoken word poem, YouthSites are spaces where young people create. The experience of creating is obviously personal. It may be supported by facilitators, mentors, collaboration with other young people, equipment and art supplies, and having space to develop ideas.

Whether the creative projects are truly original or are formulaic (even if they are unique to the individual, as Berliner [2018] discusses in relation to the genre of "coming out" videos made by and for LGBTQ2S + youth in arts organizations in California), the opportunity to create is one of the most important elements of youth experience at youth arts organizations. Previously, we discussed how the creative process often involves developing rich, respectful, and meaningful relationships with a community of other young people and mentors. The experience of *making something* is significant. The SKETCH 2005 annual report quotes a participant saying, "At SKETCH we get to create something of ourselves. People don't say 'tell me what's wrong with you or tell me your life story'; instead they say, would you be interested in learning to make this?" Just as Lauren acknowledged that sometimes saying "here's a pencil, here's a skateboard" is the most powerful thing that she can say to a participant experiencing challenges outside of Oasis, accessing opportunities dedicated to creating is an essential aspect of the youth experience. In 2017, The AMY Project website quoted Kaitlynn saying, "To make a show from scratch was incredible. You feel like you really accomplish something, that you actually did something, you can own it and call it your own. It's a great feeling!"

The examples of youth creations and creative works are innumerable (see Chapter 6), but we provide one example here from WAC Arts. The young people who made the video had been recruited for a course initially funded by the European Union and subsequently part of a raft of funding at both the national and the city level aimed at addressing "at-risk" youth who were described as NEET (not in education, employment, or training). The course offered vocational qualifications in art forms, in partnership with a local further education college.

"Circle of Trust"[1] is a music video in which a young male protagonist raps about the recent violent death of his brother and his current dilemma of trying to live an ethical life as he makes a living selling drugs trying to escape gang violence and crime on the street: "I don't rob and I don't kill, I sell drugs to the kids on the hill. . . . Who cares? . . . Life is cheap." Now he is "getting older, I stay low key up in college to learn knowledge," but although the streets are violent and tough, they contain an element of trust and security: "I got many associates but how do I know they've got my back?" The imagery is of street life and urban threat, but as the two women in the video who sing back to him stress, "For most of your life you were told to ask no questions" but "Now your brother's gone. . . . I feel for you." The heart of the song is both lament for the dead brother—"Missing you got my name carved in my chest . . . missing you bro . . . 100%"—and, centrally, the question of where he can now find trust—"Circle of trust do what I must . . . 'cos living ain't easy"—with the constant refrain of *trust* being repeated and questioned. While the author of this piece went on to achieve some celebrity as an activist opposing gang violence and knife crime, the video was an extraordinary collective effort.

The video exemplifies much of what we have discussed: The main singer-songwriter forged relationships to create the work, had a platform to tell a story that was meaningful to him, had access to equipment and training to bring his vision out into the world, and his song speaks into existing conversations about music, youth, and life in London. The performance speaks from a genre to peer experience in a way that is part of those bigger conversations, while still being his own unique story and work. Although the narrative of the song emphasizes the problem of trust on the streets, the actual artwork creates its own circle of trust. Finding the time to reflect on life experiences, to make something substantial and as finished as this video, and to be surrounded by peers and with access to resources to enable this vision to be achieved is, in itself, its own circle of trust, a defensive wall against the threat and danger of everyday life.

Conclusion

When we interviewed current or past participants about why projects were meaningful to them now or why they were meaningful when they were younger, most spoke about the ways their experiences connected with a quality of relationship and care. They spoke about the power of positive relationships with mentors and especially with a peer community. They told us that they felt seen, heard, and known. Many young people mentioned that they particularly appreciated the experiences of care, from the actions and attentive listening of their co-participants and facilitators to the availability of delicious and healthy food. Even when they spoke about the powerful opportunity to express themselves, to make art, to accomplish something, and to put ideas into action, it was couched in the supportive relationships that they experienced at the youth arts organization. Daniela DiGiacomo and Kris Gutiérrez (2015) have tried to theorize these qualities of "relationality" by reverse engineering youth experiences to advocate principles of design and organization. When those supportive relationships go awry, or the care does not accompany the experiences youth arts organizations aim to provide, young people go elsewhere.

Mel, one of the Unity dancer educators, told us that when she realized teaching movement and choreography could go beyond the surface level and make an impact on people's lives by using the art to tell stories and connect with youth on transferrable skills, it made her realize that her art is "just as valuable as someone else's degree in engineering." She told us that it was clear that what really mattered was

being there for the youth and being there for each other. I don't know . . . I'm getting emotional, but . . . I love these people. So it's cool. Everyone treats you like a human being, and, like, you can talk about your life outside, and I think that's why the youth connect as well because you're genuine and you can share that stuff.

In this chapter, we characterized these affective experiences in conjunction with the kinds of social and community values promulgated by the organizations. Our argument may sound so simple: these organizations offer something special, important, and worthwhile for their participants. Yet for the young participants, the simple is exceptional and profound. This sense of youth, themselves, suffused our interviews and the records of the sector over the period. YouthSites respond to needs and support young people's desires for community and opportunities to explore ways of communicating what matters to them (see Chapter 6). When we consider the sector as a whole, we focus on structures, leaders, cities, and governance, but young participants are at the very core of each YouthSite. In Section 2, we move from the experiential to the fields of endeavor that underpinned these organizations. Typically, education, the arts, and welfare provision for youth are centrally devised services meeting a common good. The balance between addressing people as individuals situated within a sense of collective community but significantly out of step with the perceptions of the mainstream continues to infuse our analysis.

SECTION 2

The Achievement, Impact, and Effect of YouthSites

The chapters that comprise this section address the key themes outlined in Chapter 1. Chapter 5 examines the ways that YouthSites worked to remediate, supplement, and complement educational provision. It describes how the organizations functioned as "not-schools" (Sefton-Green, 2013), espousing varied forms of curriculum, pedagogy, accreditation, and assessment. Chapter 6 explores how diverse kinds of arts practice and aesthetic experience were developed and often became identified with different organizations as signature practices. The relationship between nondominant art forms and nondominant communities often characterized the novel and original forms of practice within these organizations. Chapter 7 explores the ways that these organizations acted as forms of community infrastructure, offering notions of home and care to the young people who were so frequently marginalized and cut loose in the city. It concentrates on the dimensions of place, belonging, and neighborhood. It also identifies key qualities of relationships and an attention to relationality that characterizes participation in the YouthSites, and this theme is further explored in our discussion of leadership and leaders in Chapter 8. We not only describe personal narratives of individual courage and charisma but also identify features of enterprise and entrepreneurship in the founders and leaders and key workers at our organizations who drove their activity and success. Indeed, as Chapter 9 further explores, it was significantly due to the opportunities created by the marketization of welfare services driven by neoliberal reforms that enabled key individuals to take advantage of changing funding regimes, changing forms of contracting education, the arts, and welfare services. These, we suggest, exemplify the unique modes of governance that link together top-down policy initiatives and bottom-up community-driven agency and initiative.

Each chapter draws on the substantive dimensions of the field outlined in Chapter 1. Section 1 (Chapters 2–4) focused on defining YouthSites as a distinct field, even if it can only be significantly defined by what it is not and through tracing how its practices emerged along and across the boundaries it maintained with more formal kinds of organization and institutional practice—in education, the arts, youth clubs, and so on. The following discussion continues the process of defining YouthSites' activities and reprises some of these histories to set the context for the chapters that follow.

Histories and Traditions of Scholarship

There are histories of community arts, neighborhoods, and youth cultures, both from and about the 1960s, 1970s and 1980s. Typically, although not exclusively, they tend to be domain-specific. Jessica Gerrard's (2016) historical study of English socialist Sunday School education predates even the post-war period, although her study also includes accounts of early Black-led supplementary education from the 1980s onwards. Kate Crehan's (2011) account of community arts deals with neighborhood cultural practices from the 1970s onwards. Both studies are interested in academic work outlining resistant or complementary, subcultural, or countercultural interventions in education and the arts, respectively. Both exemplify how particular forms of learning or cultural practice emerged from divergent intellectual and aesthetic traditions. These have found a way to coexist with mainstream education and arts, where necessary, to procure other sources of funding and also finding ways to integrate the children and the community members they served with the mainstream opportunities awaiting them after they had spent time in these organizations.

In the United States, we identify work led by Milbury McLaughlin on the West Coast studying alternative and frequently Black-led organizations as forms of out-of-school and after-school provision as the progenitors of YouthSites (Heath & McLaughlin, 1993; McLaughlin, 1999; McLaughlin et al., 1994, 2009). Focusing significantly on forms of community organization, modes of community-led provision, rooted in studies of people fighting for their neighborhoods and seeking forms of social justice, these studies particularly emphasized the fight for safe spaces for troubled youth to enable forms of personal and community development on a par with their more affluent peers. Many of these scholars came out of education disciplines and were particularly interested in the ways that these kinds of opportunities seemed to offer young people different approaches to learning and to the meaning of education (Nasir et al., 2011). Some of this scholarship found articulation in the Champions of Change reports produced in the early years of this century, often led by Shirley Brice Heath, and which equally made the case that forms of arts-based cultural practice could and should be central to the vision for learning, community, identity work, and social cohesion in and through out-of-school organizations (Arts Education Partnership, 1999; Heath & Roach, 1999; Heath et al., 1998).

Lissa Soep's work at a well-established YouthSite in Oakland, California, led her and her colleagues to develop a focus on the particular and innovative nature of the pedagogy taking place within the cultures of out-of-school settings (Soep & Chavez, 2010). Bringing together dimensions of social relations, political purpose, and cultural participation, this scholarship set a standard for analyzing the interactions of young people and instructors in these kinds of contexts, showing exactly why paying attention to the quality of the learning happening here can make such an important contribution to a broader appraisal of young people's learning experiences in general. This work brings together education and the arts, while studies of youth activism and youth participation also drew attention to social and political learning with wider community benefits, although scholarship here derives from expertise in positive youth participation rather than from cultural studies, or literacy in respect of arts traditions (Kirshner, 2015).

Other youth studies scholarship has examined YouthSites in the context of precarious labor markets for the cultural industries, exploring how the forms of self-expression and training also play a role in the preparation of young people for the workforce with frequently completing and contradictory effects. Miranda Campbell's long-standing work in Toronto (Campbell, 2013, 2019), Ellie Rennie's work in Sydney, Australia (Rennie, 2012; Rennie & Podkalicka, 2014), and Craig Watkins' work in Austin, Texas (Sefton-Green et al., 2019), are all examples of interest in the interface between learning, the arts, cultural industries training, and employment. Campbell in particular has attempted to outline how the relationship between policy aspirations for employability, the political economy of the cultural industries, and their long-term interest in the commodification of socially marginalized experience, or, indeed, a racialized workforce all feed into the wide set of policy and social interests that underpin YouthSites (Campbell, 2019).

Perhaps one of the most challenging studies of the organizational dimension to these YouthSites and their often awkward positioning as forms of remediation or repository for philanthropic beneficence in relationship to mainstream schooling comes from Bianca Baldridge's (2019) study of such an organization in the northeastern United States. That study explicitly identifies a racialized deficit-driven approach toward out-of-school provision funded and led by middle-class White charitable concerns working with underserved Black and Latinx communities being failed by mainstream school systems. Here, it is not so much the enterprise opportunities created by neoliberal governance that enable the out-of-school sector to thrive as much as the need to be seen to provide for sections of the wider society who are being conspicuously failed by a whole raft of other services and a denial of opportunity.

However, the broader context of neoliberal social and economic reform undergirds Su Ah Kwon's (2013) study of what she calls "affirmative governmentality" examining the forms of control, responsibilization, management, provision, and surveillance of contemporary youth in the United States. In contrast to the tradition of critical youth studies mainly coming out of the British Birmingham culture studies tradition that explored forms of subculture resistance (e.g., Hebdige, 1979), Kwon argues that the space of youth in contemporary society is constructed through a series of mechanisms of social control. These offer normative compliance through a series of education, employment, and welfare reforms, which seek to monitor young people not so much through overt policing and forms of "hard" enforcement (not that such mechanisms are entirely absent from contemporary cities) but more through provision, responsibilization, and forms of subjectification allowing for local and national modes of governance. The argument is fundamentally that forms of neoliberal power work through a mixture of push-and-pull compliance monitored through extreme surveillance rather than through the exercise of confrontational enforcement.

The chapters in Section 2 draw in more detail on some of the theory and scholarship investigating cultural production, the arts, education, youth participation, leadership, and governance (Poyntz, 2017; Sefton-Green, 2013). Here, the case has been made that constructing YouthSites as a field is still an ongoing project, so it is perhaps not surprising that earlier traditions of scholarship have tended to focus on domains more as they relate to mainstream fields, institutions, and sectors. We begin our study in perhaps one of the better established fields of enquiry—the extent to which these kinds of organizations have created and can offer innovative forms of education and learning.

5

Making a Claim for Authentic Learning amid Changing Education Ecosystems

Introduction

The key argument of this chapter is that alternative forms of teaching and learning, pedagogy, curriculum, and educational experience to mainstream educational provision were developed, offered, and valued by YouthSites. Indeed, many of them were explicitly set up as kinds of "not-school" (Sefton-Green, 2013), where a different notion of what teaching and learning could be was the primary purpose of their offer. In the institutions that may not have had education as their primary goal, a particular vision of how learning works was implicitly central to their forms of social inclusion, participation, youth expression, and presence as well as creative production (or making, as discussed in Chapter 4), exhibition, or performance. Where institutions were established to serve socially excluded and marginalized young people, being able to offer modes of successful education was central to their political purpose in re-engaging those young people who had been failed by the school systems around them.

The first part of this chapter explores some of the conceptual distinctions at work in understanding the differences between teaching and learning, pedagogy, curriculum, schooling, and education. It then argues that modes of alterity or difference in such practices played a structural role within the versions of national education system reform that have preoccupied both the United Kingdom and Canada since 1990. We then offer a synoptic mapping of teaching and learning practices on offer by YouthSites and consider the significance of this differentiation in terms of arguments relating to an education system's claims to social justice. Three case studies describe in more detail precisely what might be deemed different and successful in educational activity as a way of demonstrating the distinctive contribution our organizations have made to transformations in learning in the three cities.

YouthSites. Stuart R. Poyntz, Julian Sefton-Green, and Heather Fitzsimmons Frey, Oxford University Press.
© Oxford University Press 2023. DOI: 10.1093/oso/9780197555491.003.0005

What Learning Counts and What Counts as Learning

The Education Reform Act of 1988 (ERA) initiated a series of institutional changes to the management and autonomy of schools in England and Wales, and it can stand as a starting point for an overview of significant changes to education in terms of system governance, institutional practices, and philosophical understandings. In broad terms, the ERA ushered in a new set of mechanisms so that a national education system could define and measure what happened in its schools. A national curriculum defined subject discipline knowledge in unprecedented detail; formative and summative, external and intra-institutional assessment procedures supported the growth of granular individualized measurement of pupil progress; and centralized financial management of schools was tied to performance measures. Together, these three interlinked approaches to schooling systematically changed the local accountability of schools; the professionalization of the teacher workforce; leadership responsibilities in education; and debates about the meaning, purposes, and value of learning.

Scholars have analyzed these changes in terms of the new forms of public management that both drove and came into being as a consequence of neoliberal governance (see Chapters 7 and 9). Together with a host of more local shifts in funding, there were more fundamental changes in institutional management—from the raising of the school leaving age to per capita outputs, national standardized assessments, and even international measurements such as the Organization for Economic Co-operation and Development's Programme for International Student Assessment scoring systems, what schools do, and what social purpose education served.

As noted in Chapter 1, there were differences between Canada and England in terms of the centralization of their education systems and different local effects at the city level. Furthermore, although we have taken 1988 as a convenient starting point for legislation about many of these changes, their implementation took time to work through. Although it is not within the remit of this book to describe changes in the school system across both countries, the first main argument we make from this introduction to the changing policy landscape is that such changes have created an extraordinary debate about what education should be.

Changes to the school system wrought by neoliberalism brought into the open a series of conflicts between visions for an education system that aimed to stratify labor for a competitive global marketplace and one that wanted to offer equal opportunity to all. The mechanisms of market competition and standardized testing seemed to conflict with earlier progressivist ideologies that valued individual voice, experimental pedagogies, or mixed-ability teaching. As discussed in Chapter 8, the adults responsible for developing the community-oriented projects that mutated into the institutions at the center of this book were schooled in different times and often brought with them philosophies of "second chance," equality of opportunity, a different attitude toward the meaning and purpose of evaluation and testing, a different tradition of the relations between teacher and taught, and the value of a community or group.

The ideologies of "education for democracy," for community participation, for personal growth, and for creativity all found their own formulations under neoliberalism. The increasing homogenization of curriculum, pedagogy, and types of schooling experience within both countries meant that large swathes of the population, as well as generations of teachers and other educators, felt excluded from the school system that revolved around test-based outcomes and other kinds of performance measures defining what counts as learning. To some extent, we think it was this diversity of debate, this struggle over values, that made the organizations in our sector so important in representing different ways of *doing* education. Their offerings marked out different kinds of educational experiences as necessary alternatives to what was perceived to be a kind of monoculture across schools, vernacular understandings of learning, and, indeed, political representations of what counted as learning over the period.

Funding, Exclusions, Ethnicity, and Curriculum Reform

IN RELATION TO LONDON

In England,[1] the period 1995–2015 saw considerable continuity in education policy across three governments.[2] In some senses, much of the curriculum and assessment part of the reform had been enacted prior to 1995 and policy change focused on the *management* and *funding* of schools. The key plank in these changes was the establishment of grant-maintained schools (known as academies) that took funding away from democratically elected local authorities (Walford, 2014). Academies and multi-academy trusts required private investment in the form of sponsorship organizations and, coupled with a loosening of requirements about teacher qualifications, initiated an explosion in new school establishments (Hutchings et al., 2017). Critics have argued that the Academies Act of 2010 brought "the beginning of the end of state education" (Ball, 2012), even though some of the new institutions facilitated by these policy changes saw a return to an older radical tradition in the form of "free schools," an example of which we discuss below.[3]

The investment required to drive this level of change was considerable. When Labour took office in 1997, UK spending on education as a proportion of gross national product (GDP) was at its lowest point since the mid-1950s, at 4.6%. There was a 78% real term increase in expenditure over the Labour period. Labour's continued spending to 2010, combined with a large fall in GDP, took spending to 6.2% of GDP—back to the post-war high point of 1973–1974 (Lupton & Obolenskaya, 2013).

Despite the pull and push of centralization and school autonomy, local authorities, and indeed London itself (which traditionally comprised 32 separate boroughs with their own locally accountable governance regimes), exerted influence over the education system. The London Challenge was initially a 5-year initiative set up in 2003 by central government aiming "to raise the quality of schools serving the most deprived areas" and to make London "a world leading city in learning and creativity" (Department for Education and Skills [DfES], 2006, p. 4). It addressed the following:

- Funding, particularly school renovation and rebuilding: At its peak, the London Challenge had a budget of £40 million per year (DfES, 2006).
- Teacher recruitment: Increases in teacher pay and a new sense of optimism and possibility made teaching in Central London more appealing.
- Leadership: The "expert headteacher" was cultivated as system leader (Baars et al., 2014).
- Summer programs for teenagers, specifically a "London Summer University" for students aged 11–19 years.

These kinds of initiatives were explicitly framed and evaluated in terms of a language of *targeting*—and in London this tended to mean groups of young people from specific Black minority ethnic backgrounds (although the White working class was often a key part of the same discourse). As Chapters 7 and 9 argue, such a discourse also forms part of the more granular detailed knowledge about sections of the population that are a hallmark of contemporary government. In education, such a form of targeting was one response to an increase in school exclusions (Parsons et al., 2005) and an interrelated rise in youth unemployment. This is crystallized in the acronym NEET (not in education, employment, or training; Hutchings et al., 2017; see also Chapter 7, this volume). In the context of intensified competition between schools, young people with special educational needs, and those marked by being "other" in racialized terms (Gilborn, 2013), became symbolic markers of the human cost carried by vulnerable members of the population.

The marketization of the school system was also accompanied by structural changes to the funding of higher education, evidenced most importantly by the introduction of tuition fees for universities. This had an impact on (the lack of) progression opportunities for young people attending the non-formal learning sector and also, as discussed in Chapter 6, on the growth of education for the creative industries and allied arts subjects (Sefton-Green et al., 2019). Yet, perhaps of greater relevance for our context here was the decline of the *further education* sector.

Although many young people stay in school until the age of 18 years, they may also attend further education colleges (FECs), which have their roots in 19th-century Mechanics' Institutes, Technical Schools, or Schools of Design, where workers improved their basic skills, acquired new trade skills, and/or generally "broadened their minds." Participation in full-time education for 16- to 18-year-olds increased steadily between 1995 and 2015, despite a decrease in funding—falling by 8% in real terms between 2010 and 2017 (Belfield et al., 2017). Spending on FEC students fell faster than spending on secondary school students during the 1990s, grew more slowly in the 2000s, and has been one of the main areas of education spending to be cut since 2010. In some respects, the growth of training provision at YouthSites can be explained in this context.

We return to the question of *curriculum* provision, beginning first with the vocational education on offer at FECs. Here, a range of British traditions collided. Higher education had traditionally offered academic study of the arts, but the incorporation of conservatoires and other arts practice institutions into the university sector meant that the curriculum at that level had been brought into discussion with labor market needs in the creative and cultural industries. Standards were defined in terms of National Vocational Qualifications (NVQs), which also underpinned the curriculum in the further education sector. Employers were deemed to be important in determining the content of the NVQs. G (general) NVQs were introduced in 1993, giving rise to a three-track system of academic A-levels, vocational GNVQs, and NVQs—mainly studied in the workplace by employees and trainees (Hargraves, 2000; Hyland, 1996). Apprenticeships are paid jobs that incorporate on- and off-the-job training and can be studied at different qualification levels. All of these forms of accreditation enabled the growth of the non-formal learning sector inasmuch as YouthSites became providers of these qualifications.

Second, we come to the role of arts subjects, and creativity, both in schools and in the national curriculum, which has been remarkably fraught and inconsistent (Sefton-Green et al., 2011). In 1998, New Labour's Culture Secretary Chris Smith published the book *Creative Britain*, reflecting his department's insistence on the centrality of the "creative economy" as a growing sector. New Labour commissioned reports such as "All Our Futures" (National Advisory Committee on Creative and Cultural Education, 1999), marking a re-emergence of arts education and classroom autonomy, which had spent the 1980s and 1990s on the margins of policymaking. Labeled a "cultural turn" in education, it addressed the arts and culture in a new way, emphasizing the importance of "creativity" to

- science and industry, due to global demand from business for forms of education and training that develop communication, innovation, and creativity and prepare workers to negotiate the 21-century workplace;
- inclusion, as knowledge-based and cultural industries were to provide an opportunity for the creative abilities of young people and to combat exclusion in a world of rapid social and economic change; and
- individual and community identity, by raising self-esteem, changing perceptions of a locality, encouraging tolerance and acceptance of diversity, and promoting self-discipline and social responsibility (Buckingham & Jones, 2001; Jones & Thomson, 2008).

However, since 2010, there has been a turning away from this creativity-centric discourse. There is no art subject in the EBacc,[4] and arts subjects are given little weighting in the school performance measure regarding General Certificate of Secondary Education (GCSE) achievement "Progress 8," introduced in 2016. The number of young people taking GCSEs in arts subject has been declining since 2013—by 2016 it was lower than it was in 2010 (Johnes, 2017)—and the number of arts teachers in state schools fell by up to 11% (Neelands et al., 2015, p. 47). Again, it is within this context of decline that YouthSites found opportunities.

IN RELATION TO TORONTO AND VANCOUVER

Many of these structural realignments and market mechanisms also took place in Canada, although the different relationship between federal and provincial authorities (Ontario and British Columbia, rather than the city authority) makes a direct comparison challenging. Different inherited assumptions about the role of the arts/culture in the curriculum, different traditions about the value of accreditation, and different political challenges—especially around indigeneity—also mean that for all the similarities between the two countries, the particular contexts for the educational development of the non-formal learning sector were significantly different.

However, the way changes in *funding* and *accountability* of schools opened up and legitimated opportunities for other kinds of educational establishments does seem shared across the three cities. The general trend of school management in Ontario was to move from a system of highly individualized school boards to more centralized control at the provincial level through an increase in regulation and decrease in the number of school boards and trustees (Li, 2015). In 1996, in British Columbia, the provincial government also centralized school districts by reducing the total number from 75 to 59, similar to the trajectory toward greater centralization of control in Ontario (Lambert, 2017). In general, successive budgets under the federal Liberal government continued to slash millions from education budgets. Schools were encouraged to open private businesses to address shortfalls, and school catchment borders were removed to develop competition between schools (Lambert, 2017).

Similar ideologies of *targeting* were evident in a raft of funding initiatives and policy pronouncements. Both the United Kingdom and Canada (at both national and city levels) are concerned with the visible exclusion of racialized minorities, but in both British Columbia and Ontario, the Indigenous youth population (as part of a longer history of neocolonial management) is an explicit policy objective. In 2008, a historic apology made by then Prime Minister Stephen Harper for those who had suffered in the residential school system preceded federal government reforms in the education system, such as those presented in *Reforming First Nation Education: From Crisis to Hope* (Standing Senate Committee on Aboriginal Peoples, 2011). Initiatives aimed at LGBTQ2S+ youth were also highly visible as part of a discussion about educational provision in Canada. For example, in 1996, the Toronto District School Board launched the Triangle Program, the first of its kind in Canada, an alternative school program for LGBTQ2S+ youth (Brown et al., 2017).

In general, targeting mechanisms are seen as redistributive—reallocating inequitable resourcing. Funding shortfalls in education perpetuated "disparities between large urban public school boards, inner city vs. suburban neighborhoods, as well as rural and Northern boards," as well as failed "to address inequities based on income, gender, race, newcomer status, Indigenous status, and people with special needs" (Shaker & Hennessey, 2018). Concerns with youth unemployment (reaching 18% in 2013 in Ontario, for example, which was considerably higher than in other provinces) were attributed to difficulties in reaching "at-risk" youth. Thus, for example, the murder of Reena Virk in 1997 by seven youths created a moral panic around "girl violence" (Batacharya, 2000), leading to a number of "safe schools" initiatives. In 2003, a new Youth Criminal Justice Act encouraged rehabilitation as well as focused targeting of the causes of youth crime while also lengthening sentences and imposing harsher punishments (Dell, 2015). However, although many of these mechanisms led to significant changes in school policy (e.g., The Safe Schools Act of 2000; see Kerr, 2011) or practitioner initiatives (e.g., the establishment of the Elementary Teachers Federation of Ontario's LGBT Standing Committee; see Brown et al., 2017), as much as they enabled targeted use of resourcing, they also contributed to a debate about whose interests were being served by contemporary arrangements of the system.

As in the United Kingdom, further and higher education were also subjected to considerable reform. The opening up of degree-granting status to private institutions as well as further scope toward research in the private sector led to a blurring of the lines between the place of the traditional university and private schooling (Trotter & Mitchell, 2018). Post-secondary schools began to operate more like businesses, being pushed toward "vocationalism," which meant the production of workers being promoted as a more central priority (Arvast, 2008). In British Columbia during this period, the NDP (New Democratic Party) Harcourt government moved toward a focus on vocationalism in higher education as well as attempts to regulate the university sector that had, before this period, existed in a "non-interventionist" policy environment (Rexe, 2015). The 2000s started out with a high degree of care taken to protect students from increasing tuition costs, but as was the case in Ontario, moves toward privatization would mean that private institutions began to proliferate and, unique to British Columbia, would result in what turned out to be a largely unregulated "gray market" of degree-granting institutions.

As in the United Kingdom, the curriculum became a site for driving school change in terms of measuring performance outcomes with an emphasis on competition between schools and standardized outcomes and, equally, a political space for cultural conflict. In Ontario, changes made under the Harris government included the implementation of standardized report cards and a province-wide curriculum. As in other areas of the world, the arts and other kinds of cultural activity were relegated in importance. British Columbia seems have endured less upheaval than Ontario, perhaps reflecting a different starting point. An outcome-based curriculum, choice, school accountability, and testing became important issues across the province (Broom, 2016). By 2015, a revised curriculum emphasized personalized learning, with the elimination of core classes such as Social Studies 11, English 11, and English 12, replacing them with a number of student choices, as well as highlighting Indigenous ways of knowing in all disciplines after a push from the British Columbia Teachers' Federation and the First Nations Education Steering Committee (Hansman, 2016). A language of general competency replaced discipline-specific traditions, such as when the Ministry of Education emphasized strategies toward greater "collaboration, critical thinking, and communication skills" (quoted in Judd, 2015).

Mapping Alternativeness: A Synoptic Overview of Education in "Not-Schools"

The accounts of structural transformation in the education systems across England, Ontario, and British Columbia are brief. We have emphasized a set of relationships between curriculum, assessment, accreditation, funding, centralization decline in local management and autonomy, an increase in private players in hitherto national/state marketplaces, and an overall marketization of the education system with attempts to develop forms of competition. Even passionate advocates of such transformations have acknowledged the stress of such wholesale reforms, and it is beyond the scope of this chapter to enter into that discussion. Our interest here has been to focus on the key mechanisms of change, which, as we have shown throughout this book, in effect created both the need and the opportunities for YouthSites. We also wanted to underscore precisely how such reform catalyzed debate and discussion about what the purposes of an education system might be. The reform process opened up space for the imagination and implementation of different kinds of teaching and learning institutions.

One approach to examining how the activities and organizations in the non-formal learning sector play a part in this complex system is to imagine educational activities (however defined) taking part outside of schools as a kind of "not-school" (Sefton-Green, 2013). This approach allows us to see the ways that learning is structured, organized, and valued in our organizations in terms of what they are not—that is, how they complement, remediate, or supplement both failings and success in the system around them because they were often devised and implemented in order to act as deliberately constructed alternative routes to achieve different kinds of goals. Such an approach also helps us make sense of terms such as "informal" or "non-formal" when applied to education because it draws attention to the way that both alternative educational provision and alternative educational experiences need to be understood dialogically in relation to social actors' understanding of what education is and how it might work in the organizations we followed. Funders, learners, teachers, students, and families all came to our organizations with notions of good and bad education and what counts.

The organizations we studied were never established to replicate the whole education system. Indeed, we have just made the point that they only really came into existence in order to intervene at a particular juncture. This also meant that all the organizations tended to have a particular kind of educational specialism. By definition, it was a challenge for them to offer the kind of total experience populations might expect from school, but often YouthSites were set up with the aim of working quite specifically on one element of the educational system because of a local circumstance (e.g., the way that Paddington Arts in London responded to the Notting Hill Carnival) or a particular kind of social practice (e.g., the way that SKETCH in Toronto used visual arts to engage with homeless youth).

Similarly, some of the organizations were completely uninterested in practices that others viewed as central. For example, development of the Modern Apprenticeship in conjunction with the NVQ standards in London offered a very particular kind of funding opportunity in which the attainment of accreditation as an output released funding. On the other hand, in Vancouver, the Reel2Real International Film Festival for Youth not only had no interest in school-based accreditation outcomes but also defined educational value in terms of preparation for and delivery of production at an "event"—a very different kind of outcome. The Oasis Skateboard Factory in Toronto designed an entire kind of contemporary curriculum around skateboarding culture, making the production process of that particular cultural artifact a way of organizing a complete educational package with formal accreditation outcomes. For some organizations, a relational pedagogy (DiGiacomo & Gutiérrez, 2015; Edwards, 2011) was the object of the project, and thus, by definition, measuring academic outcomes was eschewed.

Not only is the balance of elements from an education system represented unequally in educational practices in YouthSites but also there is a temporal effect. As noted above and in Chapter 8, many of the key actors formed their educational values in earlier times, and part of their individual motivation revolved around a passion for particular kinds of learning experiences. Thus, for example, proponents of "forum theatre," as in Vancouver's Theatre for the Living (formerly Headlines Theatre), wanted to continue to offer that experience, even the more as it fell from fashion. Forms of pedagogy tend to sediment over time in particular institutions and become part of their culture, such as London's Weekend Arts College (WAC) Arts taster-day recruitment processes.

Finally, a systemic perspective might be useful if we think of these organizations working collectively. Rather than evaluating each organization's version of education within their own terms, we can see how together the organizations offered distinct practices, clear innovation, and equally, we should stress, overlap and continuity with the ecology that spawned them. WAC Arts' "tough love" rule that students were not able to attend the class if they arrived more than 5 minutes late is a deeply traditional conservative pedagogy completely in line with traditions of discipline and practice derived from, for example, pedagogy in dance, even if the organization was concerned with developing a radical curriculum exploring non-Western art traditions. These kinds of "contradiction" make sense from the perspective of seeing how each organization drew its inspiration and how it worked significantly as a response to an immediate local context.

In the more detailed discussion of the three case studies that follow, we have thus tried to analyze discrete elements of an education system (curriculum, timetabling, assessment, accreditation, teacher credentials, pedagogy, learning spaces, teaching groups, staff structure and leadership, and recruitment) against the practices of YouthSites. We aimed to record only key examples of practice within organizations that exemplify features of education that were defined as being different from the norms around them. This is a way of highlighting the structural features of schooling present in these organizations even if it is a kind of anti-, or different, or "not-school," at that time and in this place.

WAC ARTS COLLEGE

Founded in 1978 to offer classes in drama and dance by two teachers working at a local secondary school in the London Borough of Camden, WAC (subsequently WAC Performing Arts and Media College and then WAC Arts College) offered complementary education to young people from low-income families—significantly comprising minority ethnic youth—in order to enable such young people to pursue careers in the arts by becoming competitive at auditions in London's drama and dance conservatoires. The original aim was to offer forms of training, often only available to young people from wealthier backgrounds, to develop performance skills, thus leading to classes in dance (specializing in contemporary dance as distinct from ballet), vocals, jazz, and drama. Classes were mixed-age groupings (ages 14–25 years) and, depending on the subject, consisted of between 6 and 20 students. Continuous attendance was required during the first two terms of an English school year each Sunday, culminating in end-of-year performances. Students could build a timetable of disciplines over the course of the one day. Teachers were not required to be qualified teachers but were drawn from underemployed artists and performers who also were committed to advocating more minority art forms and to working with community and youth. Student assistants were recruited early on as a longer term investment in developing a minority ethnic workforce. In contrast with the curriculum in arts at schools, the emphasis was on high-quality performance. In keeping with community arts and principles of progressive pedagogy, achievement was celebrated collectively and was marked by participation and not stratified by individualized ability. Video, digital arts, and music technology were added to the curriculum in 1998.

The high number of minority ethnic students marked WAC Arts as performing a wider community function, and within 5 years, classes for junior WAC Arts (students aged 6–13 years) on Saturdays, replicating the menu of subjects opened, created a space for families and parents as much as an educational space for students. Various kinds of school homework and family support filtered into this program with attention to bringing families together in performance, and in the early 20th century, laptops and other information technology support were available along with open internet access.

These weekend projects led to after-school and holiday projects, either organized around art form disciplines or as performance projects. As an educational experience, these practices consolidated as key leaders reflected on the success of their work (defined in terms of both engagement and the number of students using WAC Arts as routes to further progression in their art forms). The organization developed a reputation for recruiting from local schools—it did taster sessions and opened its doors each year for a kind of open audition practice. In addition, it developed arts-based activities in local youth clubs (funded by the local authority). Part-time staff worked across all of these projects, and alumni began to work back at the organization. The young people who attended traveled across London but came together as a peer-oriented community of practice. From the 1980s, there were perhaps 1,000 young people a year in regular attendance.

The arts practice itself (see Chapter 6)—forms of Black-led theater, jazz fusion dance, and jazz—also developed expertise and authority within a range of local "scenes" (Straw, 1991), again contributing to this virtuous circle of reputation, expertise, high visibility, and career promotion. The founding director, Celia Greenwood, stressed that although she had a very clear concept of a particular kind of drama educational practice and a commitment to a way of working with young people, she did not foresee, or perhaps even intend to build, the kind of experience and "mass" that began to accrue around her. The community, which grew out of these educational activities, took on more neighborhood social functions, bringing people together and offering a huge amount of advice, support, and help. As a kind of educational practice, WAC Arts developed in two directions.

First, it began to hold contracts with the local authority to support work for young people with special educational needs—including young people with physical impairments as well as those on the autistic spectrum. These projects never explicitly used the language of therapy and were not conducted by qualified experts but had developed a series of processes that were able to engage, sustain interest, and support learning progression, supporting expression by young people through the arts and creative media. This led to quite a specialized strand of work and additional progression by young people with special needs into WAC Arts' own "mainstream" provision.

Second, the kinds of practice with young people who were failing or had been failed by the school system, whereby young people pursuing arts and media-based programs achieve success and were clearly engaged and motivated, often in contrast to their record in mainstream schooling, led to the development of provision that specialized in reaching socially excluded groups. Funded significantly by European money, WAC Arts began to offer programs for young people who had experienced homelessness or were at risk of crime, teen pregnancy, and so forth, offering structured courses during the daytime. These courses were run in partnership with local schools and FECs—sometimes in a franchised relationship and sometimes supporting students to achieve formal qualifications. The kinds of curriculum, the kinds of pedagogy, and the ways of working with young people who had been disengaged from their regular schooling were thus recognized as a special way of working so that processes of recruitment, teaching, support, and directing learning progressions had become consolidated into its own "method."

Many young people who had attended WAC Arts returned as teachers often after or alongside their higher education and/or professional experience, and a mixture of core full-time staff and up to 200 part-time staff (in 2004) meant that there was a significant amount of shared knowledge and ways of working that found its expression in how classes were recruited, run, evaluated, and followed up. In turn, this expertise provided a kind of affective labor and educational experience that could then be used in a range of courses and projects. Courses to support teen mothers learning about their infants' learning—recording and sharing on early mobile phones—trapeze projects, circus skills, a Cuban music school, aerials, touring groups, and programming LEGO robots were all projects that shared the teaching expertise of the staff group, bringing in experts as required, so that students might attend courses at WAC Arts for extended and continuing projects.

By 2003, WAC Arts was working in partnership with the local university to offer a degree in non-Western art forms; this later migrated into a higher education diploma and WAC Arts became a center to accredit Level 2 and Level 3 GNVQs. It ran Modern Apprenticeships and fully participated in a range of accreditation practices. In 2012, it opened its own "free school," thus formally becoming an authorized kind of "alternative provision," funded as part of Conservative government education reforms in the 2010s.

During a 40-year period, WAC Arts thus played a significant role in the lives of a substantial number of young people given that at its height it was perhaps working with up to 2,000 different young people per year. It drew down targeted funding as well as being able to access funding from central government. Curriculum expertise meant that its impact can be traced across a variety of cultural productions and outputs. The concentration of its educational labor force had significant aftereffects. It used forms of accreditation and assessment both to drive the program and to access funding. As a community resource embodying forms of care, it exemplifies a quite extraordinary commitment to young people over (in some cases) their lifetime well beyond the "pump-priming" version of institutionalized schooling. There is no doubt that its educational work can only really be understood in terms of the gaps it filled, the needs it met, and the opportunities between increasingly impermeable boundaries that it exploited.

It was an unusual organization in the size, range, and scope of its work, and for all its achievements. We are not necessarily trying to argue that every event, every lesson, every activity was without a challenge. The point of this analysis has been to underscore how it was only through WAC Arts' institutional operations that it managed to aggregate and maximize impact.

OASIS SKATEBOARD FACTORY

The Oasis Skateboard Factory (OSF) offers an arts-based alternative to the school system and works with young people (aged 13–17 years) who might not otherwise finish high school in Toronto. Launched by teacher Craig Morrison in 2007, it is unusual in our discussions of YouthSites because it is a public school and the staff are trained and certified teachers. The Toronto District School Board has a suite of publicly funded alternative schools, and three of these focus on the needs of young people who have disengaged from education (the Triangle Program, Canada's only school for LGBTQ2S+ students; the Arts and Social Change School; and OSF).

Structurally, OSF differs significantly from mainstream schools. It is not located in a school building but, rather, in the Scadding Court Community Center, sharing the building with a gym, an early childhood drop-in center, and community outreach programming. It has none of the Toronto District School Board markings: There are no desks, no bells, the national anthem is not sung, and there is no hierarchy with a principal's office. Instead, there are two teachers and an efficiently organized but cramped design studio space. Outside, there is a skate park, which is also a good place to do spray painting, with the proper ventilation. With approximately 25 students admitted annually, the school is small. Drawing young people from all over the city, between 15% and 25% identify as Indigenous (which is high for the Toronto District School Board), and a significant number of non-Indigenous students identify with other racialized groups. Some students are street-involved or live with housing precarity. Initially, the school's skateboard focus attracted almost exclusively young men, so in 2011, Craig Morrison hired Lauren Hortie (a visual artist, DJ, and teacher) so that young women could also see themselves at the school, and school enrollment is now gender-balanced.

Through experiential learning and modules designed to achieve provincially mandated curriculum requirements, students can participate in the school for up to 2 years and receive high school credits, return to the mainstream system, or graduate directly from OSF. The students build and design brands—boards, T-shirts, stickers, and business plans. Young people learn to work with clients, mentors, Indigenous Elders, and each other. Much of the work they do during the day is independent, so they learn self-reliance. Morrison notes that the school has a lot of freedom, but "the flip side of freedom is responsibility—another anarchist, punk rock concept. We're very responsible, we're very accountable, everything's very transparent" (quoted in M. Barker, 2013).

Graduation rates are between 75% and 100%. Although OSF cannot offer a full complement of high school courses, it offers credits in a wide range of subjects, from math to English, entrepreneurship, and art. Achieving credits in high school subjects and/or completing a high school diploma are measurable outcomes, but the organization prizes learning experiences, as current participants explained:

> I think the program can help a lot of people who have struggled with school in the past and bring them up and give them something that they actually want to do.
>
> Seeing some, like actual physical things from your work is really important and encouraging rather than just like you do work and then you never see it again.
>
> Art makes you find more interests that you like.

Craig Morrison highlights the liminal space OSF opens up between participants' interests and culture, such as graffiti and skateboarding, which have been marginalized by adults and even criminalized, and the artistic influence those forms have on contemporary commercial industry. OSF students seek out clients who are other young entrepreneurs, and they start to see themselves past high school, asking questions about values, ethical practices, and the role of business in community social change.

The experience of an OSF day is very much perceived as not being like traditional schooling:

> So, start time is amazing because at, like, regular school, it starts at 9:00. If I wake up at noon, I'm not going. Here, if I wake up at noon, I'll show up for one and still have a couple of hours to get all the work I need to get done and I feel like it's a plausible thing. I might have missed something but I can get, like, caught up, and I can come here and I can work on it and I can take what I don't finish home and finish it. Whereas at school, at a regular school I'd go in, I'd miss the assignment, I wouldn't *get* the assignment, I wouldn't do the assignment.

From a teacher's point of view, that story is a little different. Although attendance is mandatory, unlike other schools, they do not break for lunch because teachers found that it was too difficult for many young people to return to class. Reducing barriers to participation is essential. Like WAC Arts and other kinds of flexible provision (McGregor et al., 2017), OSF provides many services that ordinary schools do not, such as contacting students in the morning to remind them to get up and come to school if they are having trouble attending or providing access to counseling services. But, like other YouthSites, staff are not social workers, nor do they seek to triage social difficulties onto professional counseling services.

Characteristically it is through finding forms of engagement in the work that solutions to daily challenges are met:

> Sometimes we have to pause and be like "oh good you're here, here's a pencil. Here's a skateboard." Maybe instead of this being the site where you have to come and deal with all your social problems, maybe this is the escape.

OSF promotes creative exploration and "the [entrepreneurial/competitive] hustle," while emphasizing an interests-based and assets-focused curriculum that assumes that young participants have gifts and strengths and that they need to develop skills that make it possible to control and expand the choices they have about their futures. While young people develop their own brands and do work individually, they also do work for the collective OSF brand, such as art installations at the Gladstone or fulfilling a commission to build skateboards for Justin Bieber. Evidence of the attitude of celebrating shared successes is promoted by the school blog and Instagram sites. OSF's practices ensure that no participant is ever truly alone; that even in an entrepreneurial space, asking for help is encouraged; that no one person is ever entirely independent; and, on some levels, that successes are shared by all OSF students.

REEL2REAL: INTERNATIONAL FILM FESTIVAL FOR YOUTH

Whereas in different ways WAC Arts and OSF refracted the forms, systems, funding, and organization of formal education, doing their own versions of classes, accreditation, progression, and institutional identity, our final case took principles of engagement and participation found in forms of public pedagogy (Sandlin, 2009) and translated them into a youth-focused experience. The idea for Reel2Real began to emerge a decade prior to the organization's incorporation, during founding director Venay Feldon's global travel experiences. It was born in June 1998 as a film festival for young people.

During a 20-year history, its aims have remained fairly consistent: to promote film and media education and the arts, with a focus on film appreciation, social awareness, and the development of opportunities for young people to engage in creative practice. Key institutional partners, including schools and the Museum of Vancouver, have played a major role in shaping its pedagogy and curricula. Such partnerships have been essential to the institutional growth of the organization, with the result that it has developed as a space of learning that complements the formal education system. This is perhaps most evident in the study guides it has developed to support elementary and secondary student participation in the annual Reel2Real International Film Festival for Youth and the integration of film learning with subject courses in school. The guides aim to provide forms of wider cultural and political understanding about cinema in general. Its programs aim to counter what Feldon calls the "inferior quality of films that young people [are] exposed to" by "opening their eyes" to new genres, film traditions, and formats.

In other words, its educational intervention takes the form of a kind of cultural practice, and the learning and teaching involved derive from enabling and supporting young people to participate fully in this practice in all sorts of ways. To support the Reel2Real International Film Festival, for instance, the Youth Jury Program was inaugurated early on to train elementary and secondary school students as festival judges, through workshops on film history and language, key genres, and essential filmmakers from across European, Asian, and American cinema traditions. In addition, while showcasing short and feature films about children and youth from throughout the world, it has developed a diverse range of screening, training, and mentorship programs, working with schools and school board partners and collaborating with a regular pool of institutional partners, including the National Film Board, the Museum of Vancouver, the Vancouver Foundation, and the Vancouver International Film Festival.

Reel2Real has, in the main, been flexible in regard to the young people it works with, targeting students from across the provincial schooling system and increasingly reaching out to Canada's northern territories. The Animating History program offers a day-long animation workshop in partnership with schools to help students learn production skills while exploring issues in local history or issues present in exhibits hosted at the Museum of Vancouver. Other programs, including BC Stories, bring youth-made films into classrooms throughout the province, and the Summer Film Series hosts outdoor film screenings throughout the Vancouver region. Other programs are more targeted, including the Our World collaboration, through which Reel2Real provides access to media arts for Indigenous youth and integrates First Nations language and culture into filmmaking as a way to address the past and nourish pride. Program instructors are often former student participants in its programs who return following post-secondary training in digital production and/or film and media studies. Other instructors are practicing artists and filmmakers, working between Reel2Real, the local commercial film and television industry, and their own practices.

Technology change has helped the organization shift its program toward a greater emphasis on production and engagement with new formats, including virtual reality (VR) workshops. Feldon notes that although these developments are fed by pressure to innovate and create more diverse programming, this can pose challenges to its original vision and aims. Thinking specifically about the urge to develop new VR workshops, Feldon says,

> Yeah. So, I guess you have to keep up with the changes. [But] . . . part of me hesitates with adding VR because it is different. It's a very isolating experience and the whole idea for Our World is to involve the community. So, we have huge screenings. And the Elders are listening and listening to the youth speak their native language in their films. It's pretty moving and it's an experience the whole community gets to appreciate. So [in this context], introducing VR is an issue because it's a more enclosed experience and it doesn't quite have

that same impact, but if youth want to learn the technology, it's also important to bring those tools to the community.

Reel2Real programs offer opportunities to stretch and expand notions of student voice while supporting young people's political reflection and action. In its early days, Feldon was hesitant to show any content that was controversial to young people, particularly in schooling contexts. However, as it has established a reputation with educators for caring, nuanced, and innovative programs, the programming of the Reel2Real International Film Festival, the Youth Filmmakers Showcase, and other initiatives have come to reflect broader concerns for activism and politics. Reel2Real has supported this pedagogical turn and, in an important way, this reflects how smaller, agile organizations can open space for nondominant communities, including a queer woman, Indigenous youth, young artists, and others, to nurture stories of identity, communication, and change.

Conclusion

The overall argument of this chapter is that the educational work of YouthSites can be seen as challenges, responses, resistances, or indeed implementations of the variety of systemic change evident in the education system of both Canada and England. The complex interplay of funding, curriculum, pedagogy, assessment and accreditation, stratification, progression and exclusion, social norms and behaviors, community interest, and expectation, all of which operate as discrete elements within contemporary schooling, comprised, in some ways, the very material of innovation and transformation. In other words, looking at the imagination and provision of education outside of schooling is a good way to make sense of what happened in schools over the period. It is true that the responsibilities of these organizations to the population at large were never tested, and equally, the range and quality—the effectiveness—of transactions cannot be presumed from this description of activities. However, collectively, the practices and activities of the organizations do act as an excellent exposé of the problems and deficits that seemed to be failing so many young people during this period, and which most commentators ascribe to the responsibilities of a public education system.

One question we are still pondering is the extent to which these organizations' activities can be understood as either a safety valve or a research and development social lab. Scholars have noted how, at different periods, alternative ideologies of education, such as those on offer in Montessori or Steiner schools, which pay particular attention to the way that the curriculum was organized and pedagogy enacted, were, to some degree, incorporated by mainstream education systems partly as a response to middle-class pressures and partly because such innovations acted as trailfinders for shifts in attitudes toward learner agency, teacher authority, and changing social behaviors in general (Bekerman et al., 2005; Mills & Kraftl,

2014). We discuss in Chapter 6 how innovations in art form practice, developed by artists and practitioners who were at the cutting edge of their discipline, were offered at many YouthSites because innovative practice stemmed from forms of culture that were themselves marginalized. In that sense, we can see the curriculum (and possibly associated ways of working) in digital media and music technology being trialed and tested before recuperation by mainstream schooling. But it is equally viable to analyze the work of our organizations in terms of a safety valve, mopping up school failures and coping with socially excluded groups who are being left at the margins of our cities. This is particularly evident in their work with young people from the oppressed communities that the education system was clearly failing to serve. We have shown how commitments to certain kinds of pedagogy and creative cultural curriculum offered forms of success—in terms of engagement in education or investments in employability as much as in the production of meaningful output. Here, readers will have noticed that the boundary between education and training, vocationally oriented activities, and competency (skills) development is a much more porous process of definition than found within mainstream education systems. We return to this challenge of defining a systemic function for these kinds of organizations in Chapter 10. In Chapter 6, we try to complicate the binary tension between incubator or safety valve by trying to think about YouthSites as a third option: as an opportunity for community self-determination leading toward alternative social arrangements.

The second evident theme relating to this kind of educational provision revolves around pedagogies of care. It is difficult to know how to evaluate this dimension. It would clearly be unreasonable and inappropriate to suggest that mainstream schooling does not care, but all of these organizations were explicit that a form of care dominated their practice to the extent that it was not possible for them to define or explain forms of learning (education) that were in some ways distinct from principles of love. Again, this is not philosophically original, but it says something about the commitment of these organizations to the communities that they believed they served, that they took responsibility for, and that clearly marks out their actions as being necessary in the context of a society that otherwise was being seen to fail these young people. We return to this theme in Chapter 10, but we want to end this chapter on this note because the notion of social responsibility is the cornerstone of what counts as education for our sector. To some extent, innovations in curriculum pedagogy and assessment are reducible and transferable as techniques, but it has proven difficult for us to find a language to describe this ethos of care as a separate and interlinked element existing free of what education might mean in the three cities.

6

Aesthetics and Creativity in Youth and Community Arts

Introduction

The organizations profiled in this book offer a kind of "community arts" (Crehan, 2011), "community-based arts" (Lawrence, 2006), "community-engaged arts" (Ontario Arts Council, 2016), or "arts in community" (British Columbia Arts Council, 2021). Arts in these programs, generally speaking, are led by professional artists and carried out by "community." Although the term *community* can mean many things, in this context it usually refers to people who self-identify as a connected group and who frequently are perceived to be outside of dominant cultural activities. This often includes people who may not be familiar with the language of arts as taught in art schools, conservatoires, or dance academies. As described in Chapters 5 and 7, whereas educational and policy goals focused on intergenerational or place-based projects often include community cohesion and social inclusion, youth arts projects may also focus on skill development and even developing employment potential. But regardless of perceived secondary benefits to community-engaged and youth arts practices, any study of these organizations needs to recognize the centrality of the "creative experience" on or for or by the young people themselves.

This chapter describes how creative experiences are organized, what arts traditions they emerge from, how they changed over time, and what range of purposes they afford for participants and audiences alike. In Chapter 5, we used the sector's difference from formal education—what we called "not-school"—as a way of articulating alternative theories of learning. In this chapter, we focus on concepts of discipline and rigor in relationship to arts practice, but we are not suggesting that those terms carry with them simple meanings from their formal school context. Here, the focus on difference is a means to return to first principles and to explore how arts practice acts to create alternative social arrangements as we hinted at the end of Chapter 5. We open with an overview of forms of expression

YouthSites. Stuart R. Poyntz, Julian Sefton-Green, and Heather Fitzsimmons Frey, Oxford University Press.
© Oxford University Press 2023. DOI: 10.1093/oso/9780197555491.003.0006

enjoyed and practiced by socially marginalized groups that influenced youth arts practices in London, Toronto, and Vancouver. We then explore how these arts practices derive from interconnections between lived experience, philosophies of self-realization, the role of community, relationality and, above all, the relationship between making/performing/exhibiting art and social change. Key to the chapter is the way that forms of community arts reframe the relationship between audiences and practitioners, giving prominence to modes of expression as well as types and ranges of voices that are frequently excluded by the high culture tradition of the arts in both Canada and the United Kingdom.

Community Arts

Youth-focused community arts initiatives in London, Toronto, and Vancouver developed out of several discourses and government-supported practices at the beginning of the 20th century, gaining momentum by the 1970s, diversifying in the 1980s, and shifting toward the types of supported programs in place today. The settlement house movement led by Toynbee Hall (London) in 1884 could be viewed as a precursor of today's youth arts organizations. Located in London's working-class East End and offering classes and activities in a range of arts subjects, such as music, drawing, singing, writing, and composition (Himmelfarb, 1990, p. 378), the classes were open to anyone, regardless of religious affiliation or ethnic background. Following Toynbee Hall's example, by 1894, the Alexandra Community Activities Society was incorporated in Vancouver's Kitsilano area, and Toronto's first settlement house appeared in 1910.

The early days of youth arts organizations were driven by a kind of missionary sentiment—arts were to be given to people living in deprivation—echoing widespread beliefs driving cultural policy that the arts were "good" for people and society (Stevenson et al., 2017, p. 97). In the 1920s and 1930s, Canada had a robust Workers' Theatre Movement: There were theaters creating work in Cantonese, Yiddish, and Ukrainian; poets writing in Icelandic; and people practicing culturally specific dance forms in their communities (Filewod, 2011; Lindgren, 2017). Although many Indigenous cultural practices, dances, and ceremonies were explicitly outlawed by revisions to the Indian Act between 1881 and 1951, Indigenous artists did not disappear, as the Royal Commission National Development in the Arts, Letters, and Sciences (1949–1951) (more commonly known as the Massey Commission) made clear.[1] The Massey Commission argued that Canada was under threat of cultural assimilation from the United States and should model its cultural practices after England by fostering the development of English language fine arts. Just as precursor community arts initiatives in London aimed to bring "high" culture to the working classes, in Canada, early youth arts initiatives were structured to bring arts practices that were revered in England *to* Canadian young people, thus explicitly sidelining young people's own arts and cultural expression.

Yet, the early story of youth arts blends the impulse to bring what the organizers perceived as important arts practices *to* young people with the impulse to draw on creative knowledge, experience, and interests *from* the community. Although Toronto's settlement house offered ballet classes in the 1950s, it also ran street dances, featuring the latest records brought to Canada by Black porters who regularly traveled to the United States, and these dances were frequented by Black, Jewish, and new immigrant young people living in Toronto's downtown core (Boye, 2016). The presence and interests of young people influenced youth arts programming from its inception.

Artists of the 1960s and 1970s challenged political, social, and artistic institutions, and they were, as Kate Crehan (2011) notes, "increasingly uncomfortable with the elitism of the traditional art world" (p. 3). Crehan's (2011) book, *Community Art: An Anthropological Perspective*, traces the history of Free Form, a London-based organization whose organizers wanted to share their expertise as trained visual artists and introduce "ways of creating art that would bring art's transformative power into the lives of working-class people" (p. 3). There was a readiness to experiment with art forms, and in addition, because the artists were often interested in using creative methods that drew from the young participants' experiences, the content and the form of youth arts were more hybrid and more radical than the work produced by established cultural organizations. Skilled community-engaged arts workers became better at listening to young participants, and what they heard radically shaped the youth arts sector, embracing non-mainstream arts and aesthetics, Black arts and cultural pluralism, popular theater, street arts, media arts, and more.

Non-Mainstream Arts and Aesthetics

The Appendix lists the art form specialization for each organization and shows how this dominates its profile and purpose through its mission statements. The Appendix describes a wide range of creative practices. Here, however, we focus on the main movements that influenced youth arts aesthetic practices from the 1980s until approximately 2015: Black arts and, later, arts associated with multiculturalism and cultural pluralism; popular theater arts; street or urban arts; media arts; and arts and non-mainstream identities, including a key principle specific to the Canadian context—indigeneity.

BLACK ARTS AND CULTURAL PLURALISM

The British Black arts movement began in the 1980s as an anti-racist, feminist, creative force. Black artists were making startling, politicized work that drew on Afro-Caribbean dance and music aesthetics, played with dialects used by Black Londoners, and foregrounded issues that mainstream theaters rarely, if ever, considered. While this kind of work was happening in companies such as Stratford East, the young artists also shared their skills with youth arts organizations such as Weekend Arts College (WAC) Arts. One striking example of this synergy is Amani Naphtali's late 1980s Brecht-inspired play *Ragamuffin* (updating the story of Toussaint Louverture's Haitian Revolution for London). This toured with a semi-professional cast but was produced originally at WAC Arts. The production (and others like it) trained young artists, many of whom were subsequently employed in mainstream theater and music industries. Although the dance, music, and speech arts practices were unfamiliar and exciting and encouraged mainstream companies to reimagine what arts experiences could be, perhaps more importantly, at the youth arts organization level, young people performed for their families and their communities. Unlike the early missionary-like approach to youth arts, creative practices resonated with young people's families, communities, and identities.

Like the Black arts movement in Britain, Canadian multiculturalism influenced youth arts. As elsewhere, these opportunities have been piecemeal. In Toronto, Kapisanan Philippine Centre for Arts & Culture began to offer youth arts specifically for young Filipina/o people in the 1980s and 1990s. In the 1990s, the City of Toronto got involved in youth arts programming with Fresh Arts, a program launched in direct response to the 1992 Yonge Street riot. Fresh Arts did not necessarily use non-mainstream arts structures, but it targeted Asian, Indigenous, and Black youth, making use of existing arts resources in Toronto. When a hip-hop event (416 Graffiti Expo 1999) drew attention to young people's desire to train in turntables, breakdance competitions, rap battles, and graffiti, the Remix Project was born. Initially called Inner City Visions, in 2004 it added a recording arts program to its offerings. By 2008, three Remix graduates could have scholarships to Humber College's Media Arts program, and by 2011, Remix students could earn high school credits. While these business and job-focused programs were available, the commitment to hip-hop creative aesthetics enabled numerous participants to achieve meteoric industry success and name recognition. In Vancouver, South Asian Arts was founded in 2005 offering classes in Bhangara, Kathak, Dhol, Gita, and other South Asian dance practices and instruments. South Asian Arts took part in the 2010 Vancouver Winter Olympics celebrations, creating a high profile for the young people and their arts.

POPULAR THEATER ARTS

The idea of bringing the arts to the working classes and "community" could also be seen in the philosophies of early popular or community-engaged theater projects that lean on Jerzy Grotowski's (1968) "Poor Theatre" practices along with Augusto Boal (2008) *Theatre of the Oppressed*. Mainstream theater audiences and funders perceived these as avant-garde, perhaps even slightly subversive. When universities began to take up their ideas (in the 1970s and 1980s), youth arts organizations could employ recently trained artists while assuring young participants that the work they were doing was anti-establishment, critiquing the tastemakers and bourgeois upper middle classes by making something locally relevant and meaningful to participants, helping the young people share and present their own stories.

As youth arts facilitators drew energy from the community arts movement, they began to form consistently from the 1970s onwards. For all their anti-establishment outlooks, theater creation and performance aligned very well with the success criteria developed for the youth work schemes of the 1970s, 1980s, and 1990s. Punctuality, reliability, cooperation, and presence are all work-readiness markers that theater practices could demonstrate well. As Dorothy Heathcote's influential reinterpretations of popular theater ideas became increasingly mainstream in university teacher training (Heathcote et al., 1984), the phrase "popular theater" lost much of its edge, even as funders were easier to convince. Popular theater aesthetics were constantly in tension between a desire to be (and be seen as) "rebellious," despite being dependent on state funding and being committed to the training of their artist workforce.

Julie Salverson (2011) noted that although "the term 'popular theatre' is hard to find, community projects are all the rage" (p. xii), demonstrating a shift in focus in the way these projects were positioned rather than reduced interest in their power and "the terrible beauty and staggering potential art offers, should we be willing to meet her on her terms" (p. 127). While theater practices remained the heartbeat of many organizations (e.g., The Artists Mentoring Youth [AMY] Project, WAC Arts, and Miscellaneous Productions), other organizations, such as SKETCH and Regent Park Focus Youth Media Centre, diversified or refocused their creative activities as media technologies became more affordable.

STREET AND URBAN ARTS

Since the late 1980s in London and the 1990s in Canada, so-called street arts have also been championed by youth arts organizations. Connecting with young, often street-involved youth, when youth arts organizations engage with the artistic languages of the street (e.g., graffiti, spoken word poetry, hip-hop, beatboxing, and skateboard design), this formalization of practice had several effects. First, recognition by funders of initially seemingly radical and edgy arts practices gradually rendered those arts more legitimate. Second, the creative vernacular of youth culture in the moment can take over as the dominant language in the youth arts organization. When Kensington Youth Theatre and Employment Skills (KYTES) and SKETCH collaborated to produce Toronto's first street arts festival, they did not apply for parade permits; they were squatting and claiming space in counter-culture ways. Nearly 30 years later, SKETCH engages with a diverse range of arts practices, including street arts, but it does so legally. Mainstream cultural spaces are familiar with street arts—they inform work in galleries, in the music industry, and on stages.

MEDIA ARTS

Many new youth arts organizations of the 1990s engaged with the media arts and technology. Although computers and software for creating video games, television shows, and mixing music remained prohibitively expensive for individuals, they had declined in price enough that youth arts organizations could make them available to young people, opening up more creative possibilities. As described in Chapter 1, in Toronto, the nonprofit group Regent Park Focus was established in an effort to combat negative stereotypes of the neighborhood, using newly available media production resources.

In Chapter 5, we noted how previous theorization of educational practice in youth arts organizations acted as a form of curriculum research and development (Sefton-Green, 2013). As new art forms became acceptable, so ways of teaching, learning, and engaging with the practice develop their own rationales. Photography was explored in some of the aesthetic practices of the 1970s and now has a more established place within the arts in schools. In Chapters 7 and 9, we describe the growth of Bigga Fish, an organization built on contemporary music performance that had technological, aesthetic, and commercial innovations. Indeed, creative digital media (web design [O'Hear & Sefton-Green, 2004] and multimedia [Sinker, 2000]), as well as music technology and digital filmmaking, grew exponentially over the period of our study organizations' lives and was often taught and experimented with in youth arts organizations before it found a place in schools.

IDENTITIES AND INDIGENEITY

Youth arts organizations continue to work with young people who experience various barriers to participation in the arts, and, as we discuss below, these result in creative projects that tend to focus on young people's lived experiences, amplifying their voices and helping them develop relationships and a sense of self. By the 2000s, youth arts organizations continued to draw on the previously established youth arts practices of collectively created projects, street arts, and culturally specific arts to promote marginalized voices: women and LGBTQ2S+ youth, Indigenous young people, and, to a lesser extent, young people who identify with disability and mental health issues. Alongside work with identities, some also began to engage with the neoliberal context of the 2000s, so organizations such as the Oasis Skateboard Factory (see Chapter 5) engaged with street arts as a way to encourage young people to develop a hustle, a brand, and entrepreneurial spirit and at the same time began to work with Elders to develop Indigenous content and designs.

Although struggles over identity have a powerful place in the history of YouthSites, in Canada Indigenous-led youth arts have occupied a unique position in relation to issues of justice and power. As mentioned above, this history is the result of the ongoing legacies of the Indian Act of 1876 which aimed to outlaw cultural expression, languages, regalia, songs, masks, and instruments. The Indian Act was also used to legitimize the removal of Indigenous children from their families and communities to government-sanctioned residential schools, where a program of assimilation and a history of sexual, physical, and emotional abuse left a devastating legacy in the lives of many Indigenous people. The long-term effects of this structural violence continue to resonate in negative health, social, and economic indicators that persist among Indigenous nations.

In response, the emergence of Indigenous youth arts in recent decades has been a form of cultural revitalization to support social, political, and economic goals. Within Indigenous communities, arts have long been sacred, holistic endeavors embedded in relations with the land and place and used for teachings, ceremony, and communication. In contrast to the Eurocentric worldview that Stevenson et al. (2017) argue drives participatory cultural policies, Indigenous arts practices chafe against the elitism of aesthetics (Robinson & Keavy, 2016, p. 10). In this context, cultural resurgence has been concerned with creating coherent meanings in which young people can belong, see themselves, and imagine possible futures. Grounded in decolonization, Indigenous self-determination, healing (J. Barker et al., 2017, p. 209), a desire to (re)connect young people with their culture, and to the work of imagining Indigenous collective futures, programs often work through Indigenous worldviews that emphasize "holistic interconnectedness, collaboration, reciprocity, spirituality and humility" (Flicker et al., 2014, p. 17).

Indigenous youth arts work is often combined with a focus on health and healing, including suicide prevention, addressing issues of social well-being, and identity development. These issues factor in when creating alternative arts and culture-based learning projects and processes that aim to compensate for the failures of mainstream institutions, including schools. In this way, Indigenous youth arts practices are a form of *survivance* (Vizenor, 1999) that confidently asserts Indigenous presence and futures.

In and around Toronto, 7th Generation Image Makers, the signature arts and media program of the Native Child and Family Services of Toronto, has been a leader in Indigenous youth arts since 1996. In Vancouver, non-Indigenous groups, including Access to Media Education Society and Reel Youth, have contributed to this work through programs that emphasize the meaning of the land, place, and belonging in Indigenous communities and also the role of Elders as knowledge keepers and leaders. Outside of the three cities, Indigenous youth arts work is widespread. For example, the File Hills Qu'Appelle Tribal Council in Saskatchewan administers youth workshops and culture camps in theater and arts-based practices to explore Indigenous identities while addressing youth mental health and suicide prevention. In Montréal, Québec, Wapakoni Mobile (founded in 2004) provides mentorship and training in audiovisual production for Indigenous youth, with more than 1,000 short films and 600 music recordings created by more than 4,000 youth (Perreault, 2018).

Youth Lived Experience and the Aesthetics of Self-Realization

The 1992 London-based Ovalhouse Theatre annual report stated boldly, "Everyone is an artist." This built on a philosophy encapsulated by the original Ovalhouse administrator, Joan Oliver, who, when asked about the neighborhood around Ovalhouse in the 1970s, responded, "Pretty rough. We inherited a gang, who were absolutely wonderful. I described them as creative in their anti-social activity. They were really creative about it." Artistic Director of Toronto-based SKETCH, Phyllis Novak, describes this way of thinking about participants and working with young people as an "assets-based approach." Prior to starting SKETCH, Novak volunteered at a mission in downtown Toronto. She knew she wanted to support youth creative expression, but she noted it took her a long time to develop an understanding to move beyond a service-based approach to an assets-based approach while she developed a creative arts space. Today, SKETCH begins from the promise that young people come to it with skills, ideas, resourcefulness, and a desire to create. The organization specifies that it is not a rescue or relief organization—and that young people share their capacities. A SKETCH participant declared in 2005, "They give you tools to make the stuff you imagine. It feels like you can have and do what you're passionate about." The tools and the training are offered to augment the assets youth arts facilitators see, rather than fill the gaps created by deficit. Of course, the tools and training they access influence how they express themselves, but youth arts organizations recognize that the support they offer is there to cradle and catapult young people's unrecognized expressive capacities.

Youth arts organizations significantly work from the principle that creative inspiration derives from the young participants themselves—in contrast with much school-based arts provision. Young people are frequently encouraged to explore their lived experiences, foregrounding their own identities and the ideas they care about. This principle is explicit: At South Asian Arts, young participants "develop their individuality through the arts"; at The AMY Project flagship program, young people create a play based on their own lives and stories; and Reel Youth programs invite young people to share their own stories, often with Elders, in order to foster intergenerational understanding. Some organizations, such as The AMY Project and Ovalhouse, might focus more directly on more abstract skill development and high-quality training. Others, such as SKETCH and Reel Youth, might profile creative exploration and reflection. In all cases, the content, form, and style respond to or are even generated by the young people in the room. Their presence is more than influential—youth arts organizations are ready to hear those stories and to foster creative expression defined by the young participants. It is a key tenet of faith and a fundamental principle of shared arts practice.

The roots of these principles lie in a fusion of self-actualizing philosophy, social awareness, and aesthetic value. Gosetti-Ferencei (2018) argues that imagination is a

> transformative power, which both helps human beings reveal the world, or to come to understand it in light of possibilities, and to make world, or to share the reality before us by regarding it and changing it in new ways, integrating possibilities with what is given. (p. 3)

She further explains that the act of imagining may be prompted by "our surrounding influences and inspirations, by communication with others, by worldly and cultural provocation, as well as by the existential momentum that arises from human self-reflection" (pp. 3–4).

Belief in the idea that imagination helps people reveal the world, make a world, or change it explains traditions of practice in which youth arts organizations combine creative engagement with exploring a sense of self. In 1996, just as she was getting SKETCH started, Artistic Director Phyllis Novak observed that

> the constant struggle of meeting basic needs when living on the streets allows little time for the self-discovery, exploration and growth normally associated with adolescence. Street life is tiring, oppressive and keeps youth powerless. The arts relieve the pressures of the street. Youth have a chance to mourn, express and be vulnerable. SKETCH respects the value of imagination and experience in street youth. It is a safe venue for youth to find their voice, healing, hope and direction. (SKETCH initial notebook/fundraising document, 2016)

Youth arts organizations such as SKETCH operate with the assumption that people need to imagine, explore, and create. Exploration takes time—and that is one reason they believe that the creative process, as opposed to traditional arts education's emphasis on the product, is so important.

Typically, in youth arts organizations, the "self-discovery, exploration and growth normally associated with adolescence" that Novak identifies are intrinsically connected to the creative process and creative outputs. For Ferreira (2016), exploring and using the arts as vehicles for acquiring a sense of wholeness as a person are essential ways young people engage in "arts of existence" (p. 66 et passim). Ferreira writes about youth subcultures, and although youth arts organization participants do not necessarily share common subcultures, Ferreira's concept of using the arts to develop subjectivity is helpful when we consider what the creative work developed by youth arts organizations looks, sounds, and feels like. Ferreira suggests that the work young people create most often grapples with at least one of the following three elements of self-realization: "an informal claim for a space of existence as a 'singular' ('to be different'), authentic ('to be myself') and sovereign ('to be what I want to be') person" (p. 72). As young people make and create, their creative and expressive work allows them to articulate how they experience the world and their relationship to it.

In 2017, when we attended some theater sessions at The AMY Project, young people developed work based on their relationships with their grandmothers, with their body image, with racism and transphobia, with issues based on ignorance about their or their parents' country of origin, and more. Not all the stories and creative responses found their way into the final production, but each one had an audience of co-participants and facilitators during the creation process. As an AMY participant explained in 2018, "AMY has held space for me, made me more confident, and made me feel like I can claim that space." A 1979 Ovalhouse promotional brochure, published when the company already had a reputation for radical theater produced by young people, claimed that its programs "explore self-awareness." Ovalhouse's current Artistic Director, Deborah Bestwick, explained that from its inception, the "participatory arts practice [was] a focus for empowering young people, getting them to use their voice, giving them a radical approach." Even if the creative work inspired by story sharing and exploration of the self never goes beyond the youth arts organization, the feeling that they, the young people, "claim that space" means that their voices are amplified and their experiences become more visible.

Developing Community and the Aesthetics of Relationality

During our research, we hosted several "reunions" at which we brought generations of past participants and facilitators together from the same organization. Participants in youth arts may make individual projects, but they do not create alone. In our reunions, participants emphasized the significance of feeling that their youth arts organization created a community or even a family, as when an ex-member of The AMY Project noted that it "held space" for her. Bestwick described how Ovalhouse was both

> about bringing people together by doing things, not addressing things head on as an intellectual social topic for discussion but by simply bringing people together and making theatre together as a source of debate—and negotiation—and doing it together.

This togetherness creates its own community and can thus facilitate new relationships: Ovalhouse was not just a hub for young people; it became the launch place for other radical organizations such as Gay Sweatshop and the British Black Panther movement. Although the tone is different, the two organizations established welcoming environments in which young people can forge relationships and a sense of community through their creative practices.

Although such relationships are often invisible, except to the people concerned, they are an established "outcome" of youth arts creative processes—and so are a key part of its aesthetics. Bourriaud (2002) argues that art is "an activity consisting in producing relationships with the world with the help of signs, forms, actions and objects" (p. 49). He defines relational aesthetics as "aesthetic theory consisting in judging artworks on the basis of the inter-human relations which they represent, produce or prompt" (p. 51). For youth arts organizations, these relationships are aesthetically important in several ways. First, the relationships that creative processes foster are simply intertwined with the everyday processes of the arts activity rather than necessarily held up as being "arty." They are frequently captured by a more matter-of-fact language, describing "teamwork" or "getting along with others." Bourriaud's suggestion that artistic activity "strives to achieve modest connections, opens up . . . obstructed passages" and, in particular, the idea that it can "connect levels of reality kept apart from one another" (p. 2) are demonstrated time and again through routine and shared practice. Second, these relationships become aesthetically significant in that they configure another level of relationship—between participants and their public, where "levels of reality" are often distant from one another. We return to this theme later.

Whether they are devising a theater piece or learning to silk-screen a T-shirt, the process of creation in youth arts organizations happens communally. The philosophy of each organization influences how those relationships are expressed and so becomes part of aesthetic development. Sometimes relational aesthetics are framed in terms of health, therapy, or social inclusion. Phyllis Novak, of SKETCH, suggests that this aesthetic is particularly valuable for young people who are made to feel that they are in some way broken and, as a result, they cannot contribute to society. She explained (quoted in Adler, 2011),

> The underlying assumption behind every welcome or entrance [into SKETCH] is that we just assume people are creative and that they have something to contribute. That's not always something that homeless people or marginalized young people hear. They don't hear that they have capacities that the rest of the world needs to learn from. They hear that they have deficits and that they need to get those taken care of, and then they can participate as a full member of society.

As an organization, SKETCH conceptualizes its work as "people representing various amorphic community resources who can unite together with youth to make a new community possible" (SKETCH annual report, 2005). The idea that the work is actually about community informs how a person engages with the aesthetics of the process. This is not always evident at first glance. The 2010 SKETCH annual report features images of young people playing the guitar, painting, and creating fabric arts, along with finished visual arts pieces of landscapes, paintings reminiscent of batik, a detailed drawing of a skeleton wearing an enormous Victorian lady's hat covered in flowers and feathers, a painting of the Thunderbird, and an intricately carved wooden spoon (Figure 6.1). A SKETCH participant noted in 2005, "I feel like I have jumped into water and SKETCH is helping me to keep afloat." It is inbuilt into the arts practice how producing and exhibiting these kinds of images somehow conveys a strong sense of contemporary community, and the way that the exhibition brought people together sharing commonality in the moments of reception.

At The AMY Project, reception (being an audience or spectator) included conversations around the creative work—such conversations were understood as valuable relationships in themselves. For example, during The AMY Project creative process, young people were asked to respond to prompts during their creative work as a group. The groups were intentionally small (10–15 participants and two facilitators) to forge those tight bonds. The young participants often responded

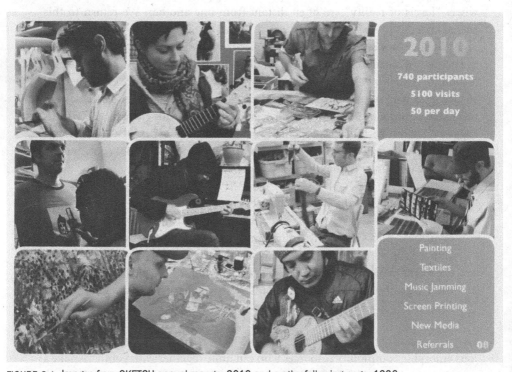

FIGURE 6.1 Images from SKETCH annual reports, 2010 and on the following page, 1996.

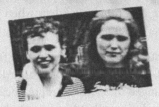

The Drug Project
Evergreen, 1994 and 1996

This unique job training program began in 1994 and has received funding and support for the past three years from the City of Toronto. A team of young women from the street youth community work together for a period of 10 weeks, using art and theatre to explore drug use, addictions and what it is to be a woman on the streets. The participants receive a weekly honourarium and are involved in workshops given by artists, drama exercises and creative writing and fun field trips. All this contributes to the public performance of a theatre piece they create together by the end of the process.

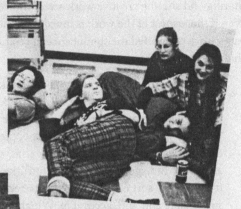

This year the project performed *Five Women NOT on Crack* at the Poor Alex Theatre. The poetic and humourous piece challenged all present with its honest and courageous look at life on the streets, drugs and the traps of addictions.

The Drug Project '96 was chosen out of 78 nominees to win one of 6 Neighbourlies Awards for its contribution to making Toronto a 'healthy city'. A 10 minute video is available if you wish to see more about the Drug Project.

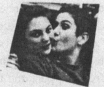

FIGURE 6.1 Continued

by making themselves vulnerable and sharing powerful personal narratives that might eventually become part of the collectively devised piece. In 2018, a participant commented that AMY "shaped me through community, through the people I've met." She wrote, "I feel more and more confident when I'm with the group, stronger when I'm with the group." Another explained,

> Being around so many artistic people who are just so free, and who are so supportive of other women, and people of color, and people of all genders and sexualities—it really changed me. I'm way more open minded, way more accepting, and I've just learned things that I never even knew before.

These comments show that the relationships with young participants matter as much as the relationships and networks they developed with professional artists. The relationships forged between young people through the process of story sharing and sharing creative work are at the very core of the aesthetic experience, even if that aspect of the work is invisible to outsiders. One AMY Project reunion participant connected the significance of relationships with the aesthetics of social change:

> It's, like, approaching art and, like, art making from, like, your personal center and your story and your truth with, I think, creates sort of more possibility and I think it also, like, in a broader sense, like, helps to humanize other people . . . 'cause it's so many different types of people, like, in the program from so many different backgrounds and stuff like that, so you don't know everybody's story and what they go through and stuff like that. . . . I think it approaches art from a really sort of genuine truth-based place that is, like, anti-capitalist and sustainable and, um, accessible. Which is very much an alternative to institutionalized learning, which sucks . . . umm and is racist and all of those things.

Developing an Aesthetic of Social Change

The majority of youth arts organizations that we examined in Toronto, Vancouver, and London were established as "arts first" organizations with social change as a desirable side effect. The primary difference between arts first organizations and "arts as a tool for social change" organizations is that in the former, facilitators focus on the art but understand that there are individuals who may benefit from support and that there may be systemic problems that need to be shifted. In arts first organizations, young people arrive specifically because they want to participate in arts-related activities. Thus, at South Asian Arts, they wanted to take Kathak dance lessons; at Ovalhouse, people wanted to be in a play; and at SKETCH, they wanted resources for painting. In social change organizations, the reverse may be the case: the arts are a vehicle for social change goals and could, in principle, be replaced by other activities, such as sports or outdoor education.

For example, Supporting Our Youth (SOY), Toronto, is based in the Sherbourne Health Center and "promotes health and wellness by addressing the specialized health issues of those who identify as LGBTQ2S+ in an open, safe, and welcoming environment." SOY includes arts programming, and even won the Toronto Arts Foundation "Arts for Youth Award" in 2012, but it exists to support queer youth health and wellness. Of course, a holistic view of health includes the arts, and the year SOY won the award, it had a youth-led zine, a writing group called "Pink In," participated in the Trans Pride art show, and sponsored a South Asian video project. Arts first organizations, such as The AMY Project, Ovalhouse, South Asian Arts, and SKETCH, all seek social change too. This aim is often visible in the content they choose to develop and their relationships with the public: By fostering youth art creation with socially excluded young people, the expectation is that social change will follow.

The two primary ways of viewing social change-driven aesthetics are through content and through the making process. Dealing with challenging and meaningful content is a way for young people to share their ideas about contemporary issues and, possibly, to shape or encourage change through the way they work with that content. Group projects such as murals, theatrical performances, and films tend to work well with themes, although the individual skateboard design projects at the Oasis Skateboard Factory (Figure 6.2) also lend themselves well to critical engagement with ideas, as explained in Chapters 5 and 7.

Sometimes, arts organizations take on an avant-garde role—working through thematic materials that they believe communities need to address and initiating conversations they believe young people need. One of SKETCH's first projects was called The Drug Project. Not only did the project appeal to funders but also the topic resonated for SKETCH because most of the young, street-involved participants had experience navigating drug culture. The project took the street as its inspiration and youth organized parades, outdoor exhibits, and theatrical interventions. Ovalhouse gained a reputation for rigorous training, even as it created spaces for radical topics. Its first play, *A Taste of Honey* in 1963, explored homosexuality (when it was still illegal in the United Kingdom) and interracial relationships. In 2020, cutting-edge projects included FiRST BiTES, co-produced with emerging artists, and Demonstrate, a theatrical engagement and workshop for autistic young people, their families, and carers. *A Taste of Honey* set the tone for women's theater, Black theater, gay theater, and radical participatory art projects providing platforms for young participants to explore the issues that mattered to them.[2]

As noted above, desire for social change also motivates a different kind of aesthetic from mainstream arts because youth arts organizations typically include marginalized people and amplify their voices in ways that the mainstream does not. We have already noted this in our discussion of Regent Park Focus and, indeed, how a contemporary aesthetic of documentary and experiential cinema emerging hand in glove with digital filmmaking offered opportunities to young

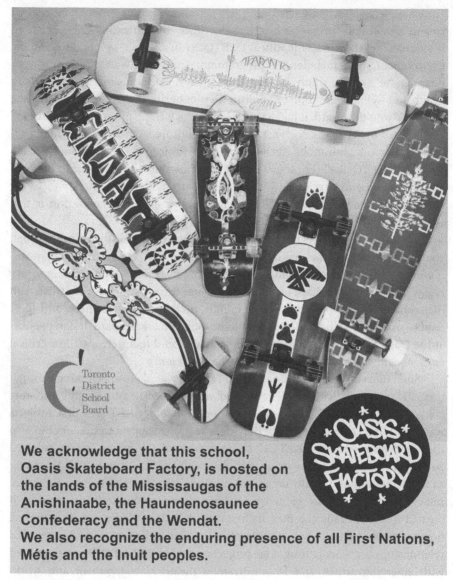

We acknowledge that this school, Oasis Skateboard Factory, is hosted on the lands of the Mississaugas of the Anishinaabe, the Haundenosaunee Confederacy and the Wendat.
We also recognize the enduring presence of all First Nations, Métis and the Inuit peoples.

FIGURE 6.2 Oasis Skateboard Factory images.

people across many YouthSites. The work they created looked, sounded, and felt different from the mainstream. That aesthetic difference was noted in The AMY Project mission statement:

> AMY understands that inequity in the performing arts industry is rooted in the inequitable systems that shape society: some young people have the privilege of private lessons, outings to the theatre, and regularly seeing people who

look like them in starring roles on the screen and the stage; others do not. We aim to interrupt the inequities in performing arts industries by creating supportive, dynamic, and artistically excellent communities with women and non-binary people from a young age.

This drive to encompass diversity pushes up against public definitions of "quality" and of what constitutes "good" art (Saha, 2017), and many organizations were keen to stress process outcomes–discipline, rigor, and judgment—to preempt such criticism. Beswick notes that one of the reasons Ovalhouse was successful was a "commitment to rigor." Access to training and resources extends the expressive powers of young people, and even if the pedagogy and curriculum of such training mirror conservatoires, private lessons, or clubs, these projects enable young people from different backgrounds to utilize the training because of connections with their own lived experiences.

Jason Samilski, a past SKETCH participant and now one of CUE's co-artistic directors, sums this up:

> There's incredible response through the arts . . . which I feel is becoming more politicized, more aware of social, cultural, and economic issues, more as some people would say woke, you know, in terms of not only, like, their own practices within organizations but also the . . . the reason and rhyme and rationale for why they are doing this work and how they're trying to pivot to make things more accessible or relevant to growing number of marginalized or racialized people. . . . So, that wasn't, like, that I don't think 10 years ago. The . . . over, about half the city or just over half the city lives in low-income neighborhoods you know? . . . I think that LGBTQ groups specifically trans, issues with trans folks and transcommunity weren't as loud or as visible as it is now, kind of thing, which is great progress. (Interview, October 15, 2018)

Public Facing and/or Outsiders

Samilski's previous comment draws attention to the fact that although creative processes can be read through an aesthetics of self-realization, the valuing of relational aesthetics, and the aesthetics of social change, public-facing projects are central to the youth arts aesthetic. Indeed, perhaps participating in high-visibility and outward-facing activities is one of the main differences in young people's experience of arts in school and in the youth/community sector. Bourriaud's (2002) idea of the encounter, discussed earlier, is useful when considering how youth work meets the public—first, the idea that youth arts from the margins is dynamic and groundbreaking, and has the potential to challenge the commercial arts sector; and second, that consuming the product enables wider audiences to somehow connect with these marginalized young people. This last idea is complex because the importance of amplifying youth voice is integral to youth arts organizations, and for the mainstream, part of the appeal of those voices relates to a desire to somehow *know* a distant other. However, the fascination with youth expression— especially from marginalized young people—can border on fetishization (Maira & Soep, 2005), and addressing that desire became a complicated management task for youth arts organizations.

PERFORMANCES AND EXHIBITIONS

The AMY Project's 2017 offering, *Almeida, the Glorious*, claims, "I will pull from my ancestors to create my new self." A review noted, "These powerful young people deserve the platform they are fiercely occupying," explaining how the piece incorporated true stories and their relationships with their ancestors, with a stage "full of varying gender identities, ethnicities, politics, and spirit [making it] the image of Canada's future" (Stevie, 2017).

This claim that youth arts organizations are the places where "the future" is revealed existed across all three cities. In Toronto, for example, Phyllis Novak described how the White arts councils of the 1990s began to recognize the creative potential of racialized young people. She argued that as result of a culture equity report (Julian, 1992), the Toronto Arts Council established a youth arts organization, Fresh Arts. This offered employment to socially disadvantaged young people primarily from Black, South Asian, and Latin American communities with a focus on the arts, as if they were saying, "Whoa! We got to break this open, otherwise we'll never be able to fulfill this rich potential that we have in this particular area of practice and then inform all of arts and culture" (interview, October 30, 2017). Rita Davies, of the Toronto Arts Council, was part of that process and highlighted the "us and them" divide, suggesting that what might be called the mainstream simply did not understand that there was a much larger non-European/non-White community within the city. Davies explained that for the Toronto Arts Council, "It was really breaking through those barriers ourselves that we had ourselves not erected, but we didn't even know they existed and we were confined by them" (interview, October 15, 2018). Novak's and Davies' responses to the culture equity report (Julian, 1992) and the culture force report (Fernandez & Fraticelli, 1994) point toward a kind of desire for the rich potential of artistic creations from unfamiliar communities. The desire clearly exists today—CUE's current website, for example, states, "Throughout history, some of the most innovative artwork has been created by artists who experience marginalization, face systemic barriers, and who have been excluded by conventional arts and cultural institutions". And although the desire exists, The AMY Project's Nikki Shaffeeullah argues that the urban arts granting system is only just now starting to operate in more equitable and inclusive ways, even though its policies continue to marginalize less established or non-White arts organizations and practices (interview, October 15, 2018). The result is that although cities such as Toronto are increasingly aware of their cultural deficits in the arts sector, youth arts organizations continue to pro- duce and present work, such as *Almeida (The Glorious)*, with a radical, sometimes startling, presence.

Public performance also showcases individuals, and youth arts organizations are sensitive to opportunity—narratives around individuals, and sometimes the success and impact of creative work. Indeed, as noted in Chapter 5, a mission for many youth arts organizations is that they not only amplify voices of young participants, but also work with *talented* young people. Davies and Novak hoped that the injection of new talent could re-energize and invigorate the arts scene as a whole. The Ovalhouse list of now professional and successful artists who got their start there is long, and it demonstrates Ovalhouse's support for new and emerging artists, along with women's theater, Black theater, and theater dealing with social issues relating to the local Brixton community.

The challenge of thinking about the aesthetics of some youth arts organiza- tions, then, is Who is the audience? Is this street art for street-involved people? Is it queer theater for queer audiences? Or is it also aiming to attract mainstream audiences? In Vancouver, South Asian Arts founder and artistic director Gurp Sian aimed to "legitimize" South Asian Arts and South Asian arts practices through public performance (Figure 6.3). The future he imagined included respect for the form and for the artist. When South Asian Arts performed at the Vancouver Olympics, it was performing for outsiders and a mainstream culture that were consuming a story of multiculturalism and imaginary Canadian nationhood, but when it performed at the Monsoon Arts Festival, it was to a majority South Asian audience. In this second case, the performance aesthetics are less about the vis- ibility of key cultural markers. Instead, at the Monsoon Festival, where the ma- jority of the audience members are insiders, performance is a way of practicing one's culture, and the focus is on building a community through interaction and hospitality.

Youth arts organizations sometimes intentionally fill gaps in programming or in spaces for creative expression. One reason South Asian Arts offered a work- shop series as part of the Monsoon Arts Festival is because it perceived a "gap" in the creative scene. There is a need for trained artists in South Asian program- ming in particular, and Sian argued that marginalized artists can barely make enough to survive—so he does not charge them for the events. Organizations such as South Asian Arts are constructed to support themselves and people in their communities. Like the Gay Sweatshop audiences at Ovalhouse, South Asian Arts performs and presents to outsiders, but it builds and creates its shows with an au- dience of community members in mind.

YOUTH VOICE, IDENTITY, AND THE "REAL"

The desire for art that disrupts the mainstream (because of where it comes from, who creates it, and why) is profoundly connected to our final aesthetic challenge.

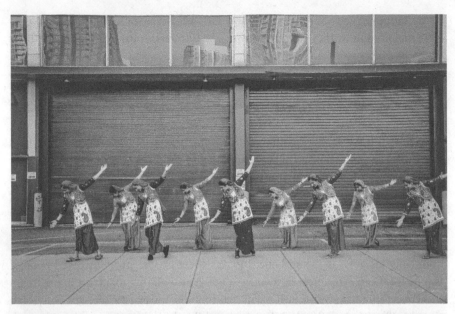

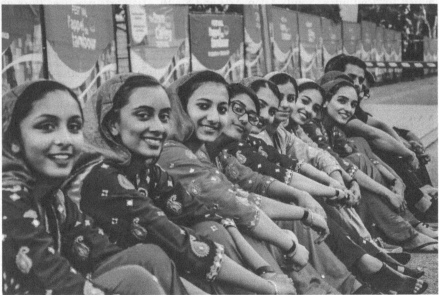

FIGURE 6.3 South Asian Arts performance.

What funders see and hear is the art. Because the art so often is created through self-reflection, the publicly shared artistic offerings can come to represent the young people themselves. Gallagher (2014) explains,

> There is a symbolic language used to represent youth, a language and discourse that is responsible for injecting particular images and ideas about young people, especially socio-economically marginalized and racialized

young people, that has served them poorly both in the public record and in the vernacular. (p. 5)

This language is sometimes present in the ways youth art products are framed and discussed by the public. Although so much of youth arts work is about self-realization, asserting identity, and subjecthood, there can be a tendency to reduce the participants to "others." This aesthetic (perhaps unfairly) promotes performances/exhibitions and so on as "authentic" but not quite art.

The final products shared by youth arts organizations, whether of a musical variety, devised performances, art shows, or poetry slams, begin as ways to explore and amplify participants—as in the discussion of the video "Circle of Trust" in Chapter 4. Although organizations today rarely indulge in problematic phrases such as "giving voice" or "empowering" young people (as Ovalhouse did in the 1980s), audiences want to connect with some kind of truth about the young people. In fact, words such as "empower" and "authentic" pepper the public-facing documents of our research, especially in the 1990s. Aesthetics based on individual and collectively understood life experiences contribute to the impression that the work young people create is "real." "The real," however, "is both a burden and a possibility" (Gallagher, 2014, p. 7). Because youth arts organizations most frequently use youth experiences as a basis for their work, whether it is performance, developing music, or visual art, those youth experiences are understood to be "true." Although the participants quoted earlier in this chapter assert time and again that the relationships they built through their creative processes enable powerful story sharing, the kind of truth existing between participants is different than the appetite for "truth" and "real-ness" demanded by audiences who are not themselves project participants.

In order to navigate the tensions between an amplification of youth voice or a fetishization of youth arts, the General Manager of The AMY Project, Rachel Penny, suggested that anything AMY creates about the young people has to represent its participants in a way that the young people themselves would support. This means that AMY is careful with language: AMY wants to point out the skills and strengths of its participants rather than focus on barriers or suggesting that "marginalization" somehow describes participant identities. The aesthetics of what the organizations present are thus connected to these political decisions. Their creative outputs can and sometimes do radically alter urban arts scenes, but it is hoped that they do so in ways that celebrate and create opportunity rather than as a form of exploitative cultural consumption.

Conclusion

We ended Chapter 5 exploring how within education systems, YouthSites seemed to offer a systemic function of acting as both a safety valve for school system failings and as an research and development lab for reform. Here, we focused on qualities of arts discipline and aesthetics to support a third role: as enabling alternative social arrangements for communities to envision themselves within the three cities. Nearly all youth arts organizations offer creative practice as part of a way for individuals to explore and assert their own identities through aesthetic forms. The story-sharing and community-building elements of that process mean relational aesthetics are a powerful component of art and creative processes. And youth arts organizations often aim for social change, which has its own vocabulary, practices, and genres. If publicly shared, these three components of youth arts—despite diverse outputs, media, and form—engage with a range of audiences: insiders, who appreciate creative work that speaks to them and their communities; and outsiders, who may perceive the work as radical, exciting, and appealing because it has the power to disrupt the conventions and expectations of the mainstream.

Sometimes, the most obvious way to discuss the aesthetics of creative work is to focus on the final projects that reach people beyond the youth organizations themselves. For all the limitations in such an approach, this matters. First, outsiders, such as funders, get to know (and believe they understand) the significance of the work youth arts organizations do when they encounter creative outputs. Outsiders may be positive about the nurturing, supportive training, mentorship, and care, but they rarely see any of that in operation.

Second, because youth arts organizations aim to amplify youth voice, and because they work with often-marginalized people, their outputs have the potential to make a significant impact on audiences and artists in the local community. The creative choices young people and the organizations make, such as their use of movement and music vocabularies, are often uncommon or at least unfamiliar in mainstream (White-dominated, established) arts spaces. As a result, outsiders may perceive the work as exciting, innovative, fresh, and new, and sometimes these practices get taken up and adopted by mainstream arts institutions. As youth arts organizations age, their work may remain as meaningful for the newly arrived participants, but the form may no longer be as influential.

Furthermore, the youth arts organizations may work with young people who are disengaged from education, street-involved, or from non-mainstream, racialized communities, and because youth arts organizations nearly always encourage young people to express themselves, their ideas, and the ideas of their communities, they connect with audiences. Among mainstream arts audiences, youth arts organization practices can be perceived as "real" or "edgy," and they may end up being exotified or fetishized, as Saha (2017) explains in his discussion of the commodification of culture. However, because young people have the potential to speak to and from within particular communities while mainstream arts do not speak to them, youth arts can reach and develop diverse and new audiences.

Youth arts organizations disrupt systemic patterns of exclusion and, as we explore in more detail in Chapter 7, can change the way arts operate in city spaces. Youth arts organizations work with young people who may not see or hear themselves regularly represented in their arts communities. As a result, the practices of amplifying youth voice, sharing stories that matter to non-mainstream audiences, and ensuring that young people overcome barriers to participation in the arts in terms of training, finding roles, and establishing professional networks shift how mainstream arts operate. Political decisions have aesthetic consequences, and the aesthetic choices are ultimately political. These changes rarely happen as quickly as the youth arts organizations would like, but by creating work in ways that challenge the mainstream urban arts community, our 30-year history of the three cities shows that change does happen.

7

Making Spaces for Youth

COMMUNITY ARTS AND THE CITY

Introduction

Distinct spaces and places for youth have been part of urban environments since
at least the 19th century. In recent decades, however, cities have regularly been inhospitable places for young people. The ragged day-to-day perils posed by traffic
congestion have allied with myths of stranger danger and a general fear of the
"other," worries about territorial crime, and media panics about wayward youth
in ways that have excluded young people from urban spaces. The development
of dedicated work, play, and learning environments designed to address the specific needs of children and youth has exacerbated the separation of young people
from others in the city. In a curious way, the non-formal arts sector has both
benefited from these historical developments and served as a foil to resist the segregation of urban youth. YouthSites have, in large measure, resisted the exclusion
of low-income, racialized, and otherwise marginalized youth from city life, and
yet the sector has also been caught up in the dynamics of gentrification that now
shape cities throughout the world. In this chapter, we examine how non-formal
arts learning organizations have emerged as a new kind of home and space of
belonging for youth amid the changes in cities since 1990.

The chapter begins by examining the new politics and economics of urban
space that emerged in London, Toronto, and Vancouver toward the end of the
20th century. As Chapter 9 then explores in more detail, the story of these cities
is neoliberal governance, which entered a period of *revanchist* politics (A. Smith,
1996) in the 1990s before moving toward a social–cultural politics of creative
cities, creative economic development, and securitization for and in response to
youth. YouthSites emerged in this context as "a gathering force" for young people
(Amin, 2014, p. 138)—a place for learning, connection, and sometimes refuge amid
the shifting ground of urban life. Organizations in London (Paddington Arts),
Toronto (Oasis Skateboard Factory), and Vancouver (South Asian Arts) have

YouthSites. Stuart R. Poyntz, Julian Sefton-Green, and Heather Fitzsimmons Frey, Oxford University Press.
© Oxford University Press 2023. DOI: 10.1093/oso/9780197555491.003.0007

played outsized roles in negotiating processes of gentrification and the discourses of creativity and fear in cities, while creating new spaces of youth belonging. The chapter concludes by addressing how these organizations have worked as spaces of refuge when relationships between youth and the state have changed and often become harder and leaner.

Locating Youth in the City: A Sector Rises

More than half of the global population of children and youth now live in cities—places where children and adults should both belong but often do not (Ward, 1978). What makes for a good city according to young people is a sense of inclusivity, a variety of activities, places to gather with peers, feelings of safety and freedom of movement, a sense of community identity, and, if possible, green space in which to play (Travlou, 2003, p. 5; see also Chawla, 2002). In contrast, young people fear cities associated with social exclusion, boredom, crime and harassment, heavy traffic, and excessive garbage. These likes and dislikes have remained fairly constant during the past 50 years, even if the major social relationships and power structures that define cities have changed.

Since the 1970s and early 1980s, a series of developments have refigured urban space in the United Kingdom and North America. The deindustrialization of metropolitan centers, the suburbanization of employment, and the emergence of global capital flows have been especially important in shaping new relationships between cities and their margins and a new context in which to imagine the experience of youth (Chatterton & Hollands, 2002).

Prior to the 1980s, industrial zones within cities were common and were often juxtaposed with diverse housing stock for workers' families and migrant and minority communities. This is evident in all three of the cities, and in a general sense, it explains why early youth arts organizations such as Ovalhouse and Weekend Arts College (WAC) in London, Kensington Youth Theatre and Employment Skills in Toronto, and Green Thumb Theatre and Arts Umbrella in Vancouver started in inner-city neighborhoods. The geography of local communities provided the wellspring from which organizations could find purpose and recruit participants. In recent decades, the ties between YouthSites and local communities have become more complex as the pressures of urban transformation have made cities more fragmented and complicated spaces.

LONDON

In London, the growth of city real estate markets and knowledge-based service industries from the early 1980s onward took the middle class back into the city center, displacing a historically working-class core in the capital. By the 2000s, a focus on creative and cultural industries, information technologies, and global financialization changed populations and neighborhoods (D. Harvey, 1989; J. O'Connor & Wynne, 1996). Various policies in the United Kingdom, including the Urban Development Corporations of the 1980s (Parkinson, 1989), the Urban Task Force (1999) report of the 1990s, and the national Urban White Paper (Office of the Deputy Prime Minister, 2000), helped drive this "wholesale reinvention," which transformed London into a global metropole (Chatterton & Hollands, 2002, p. 96).

The effect of these changes cut across older cleavages among young people. On the one hand, London became a destination for global youth cultures, attracting well-off, middle- and upper-middle-class youth and their families with the prospect of job opportunities, the spectacle of nighttime entertainment, and the possibilities of new kinds of consumer citizenship (Crath, 2017). On the other hand, the strains of gentrification, securitization, and economic development left low-income, unemployed, and many Black and minority youth vulnerable to new forms of spatial sorting and affective displacement from neighborhoods across London (Butcher & Dickens, 2016). The rise of a postmodern London ultimately made for a less welcoming, scattered, and expensive place, where youth belonging and attachment to local neighborhoods came under pressure and eventually waned.

It was against this backdrop that youth arts organizations emerged to assume an increasingly significant role in making spaces in the city. We have already seen how the development of organizations was driven both by resistance to and accommodation with the new conditions of state provision, social policy, and economic development. In addition to WAC Arts, Community Music (CM), and older YouthSites organizations, Apples and Snakes was founded in 1982 to support youth voices through spoken word poetry, whereas Second Wave Youth Arts launched the same year to develop youth leadership skills, enable youth participation in local decision-making, and strengthen well-being through training in the performing arts. At least half a dozen other organizations were also founded throughout the 1980s, supported (as noted in Chapter 3) in part by the Greater London Council's creative arts policy, which aimed to support community arts and to open new routes for young people to enter the commercial cultural industries at a time when the larger British arts scene was tainted by racism (Khan, 1976) and was struggling to respond to increasing social cleavages triggered by Thatcher's Conservative government and its policies of confrontation and austerity.

As discussed in Chapter 3, in the early 1990s, organizations such as CM and Collage Arts leveraged support from local councils, and new schemes, including funding from the European Union, helped address social inequality and urban regeneration through support for creative community hubs. CM developed in this context near Whitechapel and later became a London-wide music training program with university accreditation. Collage Arts developed on old, derelict land in what has become the Wood Green Cultural Quarter in North London, offering studios and arts training for local women and young people from Black and minority ethnic backgrounds. The emergence of these organizations in the 1990s underscored an increasing role of YouthSites as cost-effective vehicles of youth provision with sometimes deeply held community ties *and* increasing dependencies on the policy discourses, market conditions, and shifting social priorities then taking shape in London.

TORONTO

A somewhat different version of this urban youth arts ecology took shape in Toronto. The deindustrialization of the city core and the marginalization of populations to the suburbs did not happen in Canada's largest city at the same pace as it did in cities such as London. A legacy of progressive, middle-class municipal and provincial governments in Ontario resisted efforts throughout the 1970s and 1980s to change Toronto, focusing instead on keeping housing in the inner city, expanding public transit, and improving the education system (Boudreau et al., 2009). These actions helped sustain a neighborhood sensibility in the city, a sense of being from the east or west side or from smaller cities within the metropolis, that continues to distinguish Toronto's urban culture. The brutal economic recession during 1989–1992, which led to unemployment rates of 20% for the general population and 25% for Black youth, ultimately strained social welfare supports and exacerbated the city's history of racial tension between Black communities and the police. This context would set the stage for developments throughout the 1990s.

Coming out of recession, Toronto's social and economic makeup had changed. The city region became enthralled by the promise of globalization, free trade, and the new information economy, and by the mid-1990s, new centers of manufacturing, transportation, and business support industries were growing in expansive suburbs. Service industries, entertainment, real estate development, and middle-class populations migrated into the core, and new pockets of racialized, working-class, and immigrant communities settled into an emerging in-between city—areas of urban space that were neither part of the old urban center nor the traditional suburbs (Sieverts, 2003). YouthSites developed in these spaces and for a time flourished across the in-between zones and older urban neighborhoods, often as a salve for city and senior government politicians anxious about apparently wayward youth and youth disengagement. But they were also tactical sites of resistance among community members responding to racism and the exclusion of youth from future job markets and learning opportunities. We noted in Chapter 3 how the 1992 Yonge Street riot in Toronto was an especially important moment in this era, a moment that would, in fact, kindle the rise of youth arts in the city.

Yonge Street is the historic dividing line separating the east and west sides of Toronto, and in the early summer of 1992, protests broke out, fueled by a long record of police violence against Black youth, following the acquittal of two police officers charged in the shooting death of Black teenager, Michael Wade Lawson.

The acquittal of four police officers in the beating of Rodney King in Los Angeles in April 1992 supercharged Toronto's environment. Then on May 2, another young Black man, 22-year-old Raymond Lawrence, was killed by the police, leading to riots down Toronto's major avenue. A report of the province's Special Advisor on Race Relations (Stephen Lewis) was issued 6 weeks after the riots, resulting in a series of actions, including CA$20 million in new funding to support community youth arts to engage young people from across racialized and ethnic communities. In large measure, this changed the role of youth arts in Toronto, spurring development beyond single projects or organizations toward the consolidation of a new kind of provisioning sector in the city.

Fresh Arts emerged in this moment, with funding from the Toronto Arts Council and Jobs Ontario (see Chapters 3 and 6). It targeted underrecognized and underserviced neighborhoods in the in-between city, with racialized poverty and high youth unemployment. It was among the first arts organizations in Toronto to embrace hip-hop and street culture, making visible young artists of color who, to that point, were most often represented as threats in the city. The successful Canadian hip-hop artist Kardinal Offishall (quoted in R. Warner, 2006) makes clear the impact Fresh Arts had in supporting new artists and voices in the city:

> I learned how to make music while in the Fresh Arts program ... all the things that artists might have to pay a lot of money for people to do, we learned how to be self-sufficient and how to be independent and ... that is how my whole career got started on a major level. (p. 17)

Throughout the 1990s, other organizations, including SKETCH and Regent Park Focus Youth Media Centre, started in the Cabbage Town neighborhood; Art Starts launched near the suburb of North York; 7th Generation Image Makers developed to reach Indigenous youth; and Arts for Children and Youth (now Vibe Arts) launched in Old Toronto. Figure 7.1 shows the location of groups in the in-between city, highlighting the growth of low-income, racialized communities beyond Toronto's city core, in neighborhoods historically lacking access to public transit and other resources. YouthSites emerged in these zones as spaces to bring people together and, as discussed in Chapter 6, to create community, explicitly to mitigate the effects of spatial sorting and to connect racialized, marginalized youth with social opportunity.

Although community arts had a history to this point in Toronto, by the 1990s arts and cultural practices were seen as new tools for managing youth alienation, while stitching youth ambitions to changing job markets. In a real sense, these actions made communities of socially marginalized youth visible to the urban elite, often for the first time. Rita Davies, Executive Director of the Toronto Arts Council from 1984 to 1999, made this point in an interview:

> It was our understanding that there was a need and that it hadn't even been seen before, never mind being articulated—I mean it was certainly understood

THE SOCIAL GEOGRAPHY OF TORONTO

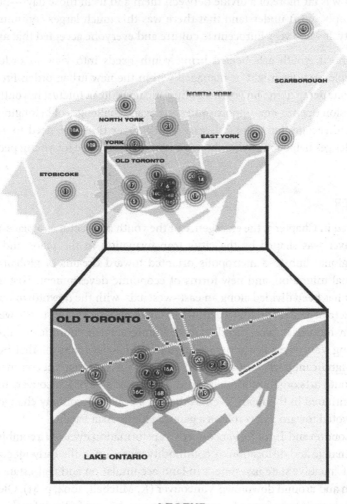

LEGEND

1	7th Generation Toronto	9	Scarborough Arts	16A	SKETCH Working Arts - QSpadina Ave
2	Artheart	10A	UrbanArts - John St	16B	SKETCH Working Arts - King St
3	Art Starts Toronto	10B	UrbanArts - Bartonville Ave	16C	SKETCH Working Arts - Shaw St
4	Children's Peace Theatre	11	Arts Etobicoke	17	Talk to Youth Lately/Looup Theatre
5	CUE	12	Nia centre for the arts	18	The AMY Project
6	Kapisanan Philippine Centre for arts and culture	13	Oasis Skateboard Facotry	19	The REMIX Project (former, Inner City Visions)
7	KYTES	14	Regent Park Focus Media Arts Centre	20	SOY (Supporting Our Youth)
8	Lakeshore Arts	15	RISE Edutainment	21	Young People's Press

FIGURE 7.1 Map of old Toronto: locations of groups in the in-between city.

Diagram designed by Lachlan Stewart compiled from locations on Google Maps in the communities themselves, but—in what you might call the mainstream, which was far more of a divide between them and us in those days—because we simply didn't understand that there was this much larger community in the city. It was a very Eurocentric culture and everyone accepted that as such.

In this context, youth arts helped bring youth needs into view in order that young people's actions might be managed within the new urban order. From the organization's perspective, however, funding streams and an interest in youth creative expression opened new opportunities to engage challenges of belonging, connection, and recognition among diverse youth. Over time, the need to address these challenges helped make YouthSites a new kind of home for young people in Toronto.

VANCOUVER

As discussed in Chapter 3, the emergence of the youth arts sector as a place-maker in Vancouver was shaped by the city's transformation in the 1980s and 1990s from a regional hub to a metropolis oriented toward dreams of globalization, international migration, and new forms of economic development. Historically, Vancouver has been divided along an east–west axis, with the downtown business and commercial area separating wealthy tree-lined neighborhoods to the west and north from industrial, working-class, and immigrant communities in the east. Surrounding Vancouver is a series of largely middle-class suburbs that have always had significant pockets of racialized, low-income, and migrant communities. The first youth arts organizations emerged on the east side of Vancouver, and this pattern continued in the 1990s, even as the city's political economy changed and the city pivoted toward a new role as a gateway to the Asia Pacific.

Like London and Toronto, Vancouver's transformation involved a combination of spatial change and dislocation. A commodity recession in the early 1980s led to a period of "massive state investment in land accumulation and real-estate development" in and around downtown Vancouver (K. Mitchell, 2004, p. 41). Older industrial lands were transformed into sites for spectacles and festivals for the global elite (e.g., the 1986 World Exposition, known locally as Expo '86, and, later, the 2010 Winter Olympics), a process followed in turn by the privatization, rezoning, and marketing of large swathes of downtown property to offshore developers from Hong Kong. A period of gentrification and social dislocation followed.

In practical terms, the migration of professionals, care industry workers, and artists into the downtown and east Vancouver areas led to a rise in real estate values and the slow outward migration of working-class and lower income people to suburban pockets around the city (Danyluk & Ley, 2007; Phillips-Watts et al., 2005). Meanwhile, new employment clusters developed downtown aided by the rezoning of the inner city under the guise of the "Vancouver Central Area Plan" (Vancouver City Council, 1991), the most important strategic policy initiative in the post-war era in Vancouver (Murray & Hutton, 2012). By the late 1990s, a knowledge-intensive economy came to dominate the city, fueled by vast real estate speculation and creative industries growth.

In this context, as in London and Toronto, YouthSites became strategic and tactical responses to change in Vancouver. The development of youth arts organizations in the city, including The Cinémathèque's Education programs, YouthCo HIV & Hep C Society, Check Your Head, the Purple Thistle Centre, and Miscellaneous Productions, was aided by state project funding meant to empower youth, protect teens from violence, foster skills development, and support the creation of youth spaces. But this support emerged just as Canada's social safety net and community recreational infrastructures fell into decline (Browne, 2003; Coles, 2007). New partnerships with local, nonprofit groups thus enabled governments to acknowledge the power of the arts as a vehicle for social belonging and personal growth while extending or sustaining state oversight of potentially troublesome youth through cost-effective partnerships (Ilcan & Basok, 2004; Poyntz, 2018).

Rather than following youth to underserviced city margins, much of the sector developed in the 1990s in and around the downtown and east side of the city. The Cinémathèque, Purple Thistle Institute, Miscellaneous Productions, YouthCo, and Check Your Head all launched in downtown and east Vancouver, among congregations of artists and cultural workers (who often found work with organizations) and within reasonable proximity of historically low-income, racialized neighborhoods. We noted in Chapter 3 that the Gulf Islands Film & Television School launched on Galiano Island, a small community just offshore from Vancouver. Among all these groups, a strong political sensibility dominated and drew inspiration from HIV/AIDS-related cultural activism, a legacy of social movements, alternative media and arts communities, and a history of alternative lifestyles in Vancouver. These sensibilities informed the mandates of youth arts organizations as sites of empowerment but also as places of refuge and welcome.

By the mid-1990s, a nascent "sector" had turned a corner of sorts in each of the cities, growing from a series of occasional groups and projects to become a mode of provision for learning, expression, and connection. The rise of the youth arts sector in cities at the end of the 20th century was fueled in part by changes in the political economy of urban space. But, as discussed in Chapter 4, it was also a consequence of a set of tactical acts by organization leaders, funders, and sometimes youth. As sites of training and belonging, YouthSites offered youth access to arts and culture through equal measures of mentoring, care, nutrition, and connection. In this way, although not a home in some traditional sense, YouthSites were increasingly doing the kind of "border work" associated with home (Christensen & O'Brien, 2003, p. 4), helping young people find ground and orient to the world beyond them (Poyntz, 2021). Paddington Arts in London is a good example:

> Paddington Arts is a family and a community. . . . We're definitely into the second generation of Paddington Arts members. People who come here as children are now grown up and bringing their children to Paddington Arts.

And if I think of anything as a measure of success, I would put that very high. (quoted in Paddington Arts 20th Anniversary Reunion, 1987–2007)

We suggest YouthSites helped resist and counter young people's experience of isolation and dislocation from community, serving as spaces of re-traditionalization (Beck, 1992) in a context of radical change and social fragmentation. Moving into the new millennium, YouthSites had come to function as home bases enabling youth to discover external relationships, negotiate identities and social skills, and develop routes toward possible futures.

From Care to Creativity

Across the three cities, the 2000s marked a period of growth, transition, and, in some instances, decline in the youth arts sector. Among the forces driving this process, new social–cultural politics of creative cities and creative economic development cast YouthSites in a different light. These developments brought new opportunities for funding and partnerships, while accelerating the challenges of gentrification, marketization, and the securitization of youth. The work of Richard Florida (2002) on creative economic development has been central to this drama and has shaped policies that in one way or another have been prominent in all three of the cities. Central to Florida's influence has been his contention that arts and culture offer mechanisms of urban economic development that can serve to rebrand cities and attract talent, investment, and tourism in a time of intensive global competition (Leslie & Hunt, 2013). These arguments extend a logic of neoliberalism: Arts and culture are instrumentalized and put in the service of economic growth. The resulting "culture–economic paradigm" casts new light on YouthSites, highlighting the significance of youth training in the arts for access to job markets, even as it narrows the role organizations might play in the lives of youth (Russo & van der Borg, 2010, p. 668). The effects of this culture–economic paradigm were compounded by a parallel anxiety about urban security and young people: In order for culture and cosmopolitanism to thrive, safety, security, and the cleansing of the city are required. In this context, the youth arts sector occupies a complex role, a node of security and often support amidst urban environments being shaped by creative cities discourses, the global financial crisis, and the subsequent period of austerity and transition that has challenged the place of young people in cities. Three organizations in London, Toronto, and Vancouver highlight this trajectory.

PADDINGTON ARTS

London's Paddington Arts started out as the Paddington Farm Trust in the 1980s, and the program's early success at teaching inner city youth documentary filmmaking led to a series of TV pieces (such as the 1987 series, *Running Loose*).

With support from the (now defunct) Inner-City London Education Authority, Paddington Arts moved into a rundown building in Westminster in 1990, and eventually acquired funds from the National Lottery, the New Labour government, and other sources to build a new centre. The new performing arts and culture center for young people opened in 1998, and the recent history of the organization and the building (Figure 7.2) show how the work of place-making by YouthSites has changed in recent years.

Located on the edge of what had historically been a low-income, Afro-Caribbean neighborhood in the Notting Hill area of West London, Paddington Arts has long drawn from local participants, acting as a gathering place in the midst of a region undergoing massive waves of gentrification. In the late 1990s, the area around the arts centre, the local authority of Westminster, included two of London's poorest postal districts, despite extremes of neighboring affluence. Paddington Arts has regularly drawn a high percentage of participants from low-income groups, Black and minority ethnic communities, and single-parent families. The relationship between Paddington Arts and the local community has of course changed in recent years, but even in 2009 and 2010, of 568 student participants, 79% came from minority ethnic groups, and 15% had a disability (Paddington Arts Report into Performing Arts and Media, 2011).

In this context, Paddington Arts' programming aimed to remove barriers to participation in the arts by offering "a safe, friendly and fully accessible building" (Paddington Arts Business Plan, 2002–2005). Within its open-access structure, it helped young people

> increase their creative . . . skills and powers of self-expression; . . . dismantle cultural, physical, economic and attitudinal barriers to the arts; . . . [and] work with partners in the community to maximize the take-up of . . . programs and the use of [Paddington Arts'] facilities. . . . [Paddington Arts also aims to] contribute to the economics, environmental and social regeneration of [the] immediate community. (Paddington Arts Developmental Plan, 1998–2001)

This work reflects its role as a site of place-making through the arts. Between the mid-2000s and 2015, street dance became an essential focus of this work, with particular strengths in b-boy (breaking or breakdance) training and showcases for all genders:

> The main dance style we do is "street dance," because this is where popular culture is at. Street dance and youth culture in general is largely influenced by Black American culture which includes music, dance and fashion, which of course has roots in Africa and the Caribbean. Black British kids have similar cultural roots, so the dance styles they grow up with, both in their homes and on television, are the basis for shared cultural experiences which we acknowledge and help develop. (Paddington Arts 20th Anniversary Reunion, 1987–2007)

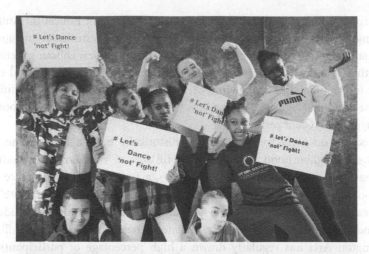

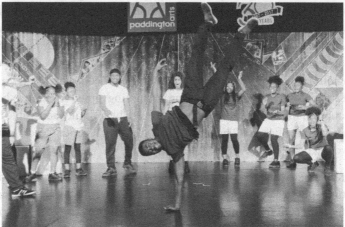

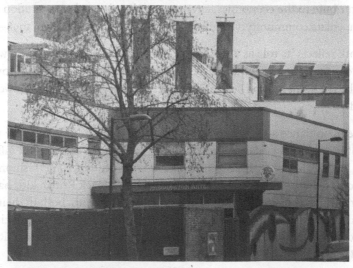

FIGURE 7.2 Paddington Arts building and performances.

Consistent with this work, since 2005 Paddington Arts has produced a series of workshops to support youth participation in the Notting Hill Carnival, the largest street festival in Europe and one of the most important celebrations of Afro-Caribbean culture throughout the world. Through its Teen Talk series, it has also engaged with social issues in the city, including homelessness and gang cultures in London.

In this way, Paddington Arts has become a destination and presence in Westminster. It occupies and operates as a place in the community, a position that was cemented with the purchase and renovation of its building. Steve Shaw, long-time Executive Director of Paddington Arts, explains:

> The purchase of the building . . . establish[ed] long term security for the organization and its activities. The acquisition and improvement of the building . . . provide[d] the organization with an asset base as well as a secure home. It also increase[d] secure self-generated income from permanent lettings of the space. (Paddington Arts Business Plan, 1995)

Having space has been valuable for the organization as well as providing a destination in the neighborhood, a site of community connection and gathering, even as creative space has become subject to intense forms of marketization and exclusiveness throughout London.

For the most part, the state's concern for the creative industries, or what we have called the culture–economic paradigm in the United Kingdom, led to policies focused on the development of London as a leading creative, entrepreneurial, global city. Development of powerful technology centers, strong cultural industries, and an entrepreneurial youthfulness linked to hi-tech start-ups, young artists, fashion designers, and other creatives were all part of this agenda (Butcher & Dickens, 2016). So, too, was a new emphasis on cosmopolitanism and cultural diversity, both of which were seen as resources to rebrand cities and neighborhoods as hubs of creativity and welcome. Amid the concern for new opportunity, however, this period also witnessed renewed concern for the regulation of unemployed, unengaged, and otherwise socially marginalized youth. New categories emerged or were popularized, including the term CHAV (council housed and violent) and the acronym NEET (not in education, employment, or training) to represent socially marginalized youth. In general, mainstream media continued to underrepresent minority youth, and when represented at all, media discourses tended to focus attention on stories of immigration, terrorism, and crime (Firmstone et al., 2019). In this context, the significance of youth arts organizations was both amplified and challenged.

In the 2000s, New Labour's interest in the arts, young people, and cultural regeneration created new funding opportunities for YouthSites. In the case of Paddington Arts, Shaw suggests that the resulting state and National Lottery funds and related support were crucial for the organization's development: "It was a Labour agenda that we benefited from and I was very happy to have the discussions about social inclusion, cultural diversity, community cohesion. . . . [We] were involved in developing policy" (Interview with Steve Shaw and Eldora Edward, Paddington Arts). As a creative economic mandate enabled Paddington Arts to grow, New Labour's concern for social inclusion simultaneously fed the interests of organizations such as Paddington Arts by opening up new lines of funding linked to social regeneration and support for racially marginalized youth. By 2005 and 2006, project funding to address vulnerable youth populations comprised approximately 60% of its income, helping the organization use its space to engage youth and make "the reality of inequality and poverty *visible*" (Smithsimon, 2010, p. 718). Yet, at the same time, New Labour's interest in creative cities compounded the problems of gentrification and social dislocation that Paddington Arts and other youth arts groups responded to. In the Westminster area of London, for instance, the winnowing away of Housing Benefit alongside the gentrification of the West End pushed local residents out of the area, leading to the out-migration of "over 1,000 families" by 2012 (Paddington Arts annual report, 2012–2013).

Even amidst this change, however, Paddington Arts created a site for the community to see itself and be seen by others. This has been most evident in its successful collaboration with the Notting Hill Carnival from the late 1990s to the present. Carnival combines the allure of creative arts and dance with the spectacle of celebration. For Paddington Arts, the Carnival has been both "a high-profile sign that Paddington Arts continues to produce top quality work and . . . a way of maintaining strong links within the wider community (Paddington Arts Business Plan, 2006–2009). Street festivals, such as Notting Hill Carnival in London and Caribana Festival in Toronto, have been criticized for the way they can represent the Disneyfication of culture, a homogenization of "ethnocultural differences" that strip cultures of their "difficult aspects" to make them safe for mass consumption (Taucar, 2016, p. 3). However, Paddington Arts' history of work suggests to us that ethnocultural festivals can also operate within a larger cultural and urban context.

The street can be a performative, social space that can serve equally "as a tool of thought and of action" (Lefebvre, 1991, p. 26). Street-centered activity is something institutions, including the state, the police, and other forces of regulation, try to control and securitize. Because of this, street performances and street festivals often represent difficult and stressful urban conditions (Sennett, 2017)—instances in which diverse communities appear together, sometimes in ways that resist disciplinary power, including that of the state. Jacqui Taucar (2016) offers a history of the street as stage, marking the way Toronto's Caribana Festival, Fringe Theatre festivals, and other events and traditions have turned the street into a platform for the negotiation and rearticulation of identities and social and political action. In London, Carnival performed this sort of function and in ways noted by a group of longtime Paddington Arts members:

STEVE SHAW: When you say, "Power to the people," the people have the
power at Carnival. It's not controlled by anybody. Not by government,

not by any one person. It's there because people want to represent
themselves.

PAT: There are people who want to take Carnival away from the people
because they think that Carnival is too successful. But the community of
Carnival has been very resilient in still having it going. That resilience is
the same with Paddington Arts.

STEVE SHAW: We are happy to be part of Carnival because it's again about
sharing values, about creativity, community spirit, supporting each
other, working together . . . all those things that we feel sometimes the
government is sometimes trying to crack down and not let us have fun
and keep us down and oppress us. For those 2 days, people can express
themselves.

New Labour's desire to align with "authentic" street cultures that have global consumer appeal, including hip-hop and street dance, helped route funding and support for events like Carnival and youth arts organizations like Paddington Arts
and Bigga Fish (see Chapter 9), which staked their credibility on providing minority ethnic youth with training for cultural industries. But public celebrations
such as Carnival also claim public space by those not always welcome in public. In
this way, Paddington Arts' association and participation in Carnival have marked
it as a political organization—a site of place-making that serves to strengthen
community belonging and identity.

Similarly, by giving youth cameras to document homelessness and life on the
streets, Paddington Arts has been able to channel the state's interest in youth experience and voice into political expressions about how and for whom space is used
and the forces serving to dislocate young people and their families from community. Among their most recent programs, *Streetlife* uses spoken word, dance,
and photography to examine what it means to be a teenager today: "[Streetlife
looks] at issues such as living on the streets; drugs; families living under stress;
and the need to fit in and feel part of something" (Paddington Arts annual report,
2016–2017). Local spaces, including food shops, alleyways, building fronts, and
council housing, are featured with stories of young people working to find a sense
of belonging and home while shuffling through foster care networks, moving
apartments, and surviving family traumas (Figure 7.3).

State support for Paddington Arts and other youth arts organizations peaked
during the first decade of the 2000s (annual reports 2012–2013 and 2016–2017).
Following the global financial crisis in 2008 and the election of a Conservative government in the United Kingdom in 2010, the subsequent contraction in state support for a creative cities agenda, amidst a general policy environment focused on
austerity, has been especially challenging. Paddington Arts' funding has declined
by more than 33% since 2011, and much of its remaining support has come from
third party sources or from funds it has generated from building rentals and associated fee-for-service work. The spatial politics of the organization are no less

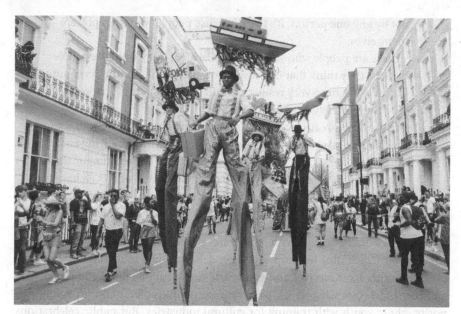

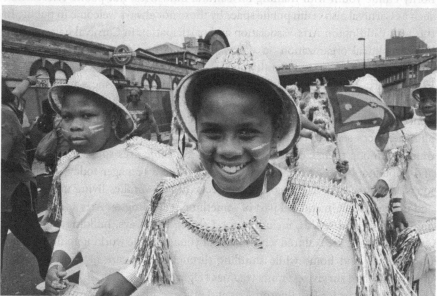

FIGURE 7.3 Carnival images from Paddington Arts annual report.

relevant, but the means to support a tactical use of space in the neighborhood
have changed as communities have dispersed with rising real estate costs and
support for local housing estates reaching crisis levels—evidenced most spectac-
ularly by the infamous Grenfell Tower fire in 2017, a tragedy that broke out just to
the west of Paddington Arts in North Kensington.

OASIS SKATEBOARD FACTORY

While London's YouthSites sector was expanding at the end of the 20th century, the wave of development across the sector in Toronto at that time came to a crashing halt with the election of a Conservative provincial government in 1995 under Mike Harris (Parris, 2018). The subsequent amalgamation of the Municipality of Toronto with its six surrounding suburban municipalities as a cost-saving measure early in 1998 reshaped the politics of the city and the youth arts sector. The Conservative government's so-called Common Sense Revolution exacerbated divisions as the amalgamation of Toronto shifted power to the merged suburbs, leaving the older city core and the in-between city with notably less representation at provincial and municipal levels (Boudreau et al., 2009). This left the in-between city devoid of key resources, even as the needs of low-income, racialized communities grew.

The youth arts sector gained ground in this context, evidenced by the launch and/or expansion of nearly a dozen organizations in the post-2000s era. The so-called 'Summer of the Gun' (see Chapter 8) in Toronto in 2005 intensified calls for community support. The shooting of 26 young men (50% of all gun-related homicides that year), largely from Black and immigrant backgrounds, between June and September 2005 led "public and private funders . . . to back arts-based community programs" (Parris, 2018, para. 6) to support the development of youth job skills and training for the arts and culture industries. The Graffiti Transformation Project (GTP) started in this context, and it exemplifies tensions that became endemic to how youth arts were supported in Toronto.

The GTP originated in 1996 as a moralizing safety-oriented directive that recognized street art as a global youth form with popular and commercial appeal, even while it attempted to direct youth expression and behavior away from graffiti toward state-funded service agencies. From 2004 to 2011, the second phase of the program (Figure 7.4) shifted to "funding projects in economically and socially disenfranchised inner-city and inner-suburban areas of Toronto," with the aim of funding "graffiti abatement and mural creation initiatives" in the service of a safe streets and a creative cities agenda (Crath, 2017, pp. 1263–1264). Rory Crath (2017) notes that as much as the GTP opened up "new possibilities" for shaping the community's relationship with public space, the program also acted as an instrument for "visualizing and rendering intelligible inner city, suburban, racialized youth" and the community spaces targeted for transformation (p. 1264). The GTP is, of course, only one program, but it marked an expansive effort—epitomized by the creation of the Toronto Arts Foundation Arts for Youth Award in 2007—by the City of Toronto to use youth arts as a way to identify, recruit, and, in a sense, manage youth populations in the city.

Among the organizations that emerged in this context, most groups (Kapisanan, CUE, Children's Peace Theatre, Unity Charity, RISE Edutainment, and Artists Mentoring Youth Project) set up in neighborhoods in the in-between city, either in regions surrounding the downtown core of Toronto or in low-income

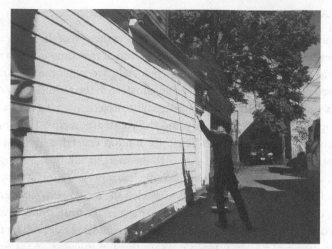

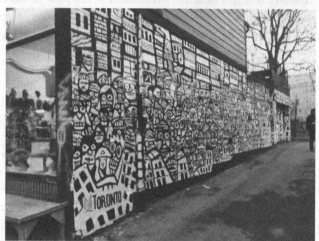

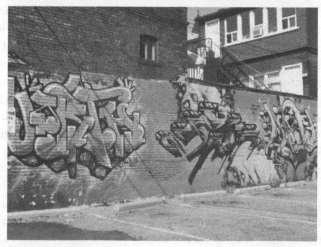

FIGURE 7.4 GTP images, graffiti.

neighborhoods in suburban ring regions of the city. A selection of organizations also focused on drawing youth back into the city by, among other things, offering food and transit tokens and leveraging the allure of street art, hip-hop, and skateboard culture to develop cool, welcoming youth destinations. The widely successful Remix Project (see Chapter 3) showcases a strong commercial dimension to these projects. Relatedly, Oasis Skateboard Factory (OSF) highlights how organizations have used a language of creativity, branding, and training for commercial success, even while attempting to negotiate and reinvigorate public spaces for young people in Toronto.

As discussed in Chapter 5, OSF emerged in 2007 as an alternative-to-school design program in a space in Scadding Court Community Center in a historically low-income, immigrant-centered neighborhood in Toronto. Participants are aged 16–18 years and earn high school credits over one or two semesters by creating their own brands and running a professional skateboard/design company. The program is an extension of the Toronto District School Board, but it has all the markings of a youth arts program, operating outside the normal strictures of formal schooling in a flexible space that resembles a design studio as much as a classroom.

Its appeal is largely anchored around the allure of entrepreneurialism, the aura of the creative artist, and the prospect of work in the creative economy. The street and specific forms of public space are presented as route and stage for social futures. OSF draws on and uses various urban spaces and its own rich networks in the city as places and curriculum resources for learning. Strategically, it offers a gateway to engage local business networks; alternative production associations; celebrity allies, including Shepard Fairey and Mark Titchner (artists who bridge divides between street/public art and graffiti cultures); and inner city arts communities, including Queen Street West and Kensington Market in Toronto. OSF trades in the appeal of hidden spaces for youth, including sites such as

> [one] tucked down a dumpster-blocked laneway off of Dufferin . . . [where] the Oasis Skateboard Factory Pop-Up was a-buzz with participating student entrepreneurs, supportive friends and family, Toronto Design Offsite attendees and maybe one or two lured in with the promise of free Glory Hole Doughnuts [an upmarket Toronto shop offering traditional and artisanal fair]. (Oasis Skateboard Factory, 2013)

OSF also trades in the appeal of the street and related spaces—a skate park, a nontraditional classroom, the side of a building—as expressions of youth autonomy and community (Figure 7.5).

To support their work, OSF has made significant efforts to engage urban Indigenous communities, including knowledge-keepers and Elders from local and more distant regions, who carry forms of wisdom excluded from mainstream schooling. Tactically, OSF addresses young people as participants in the city, actors

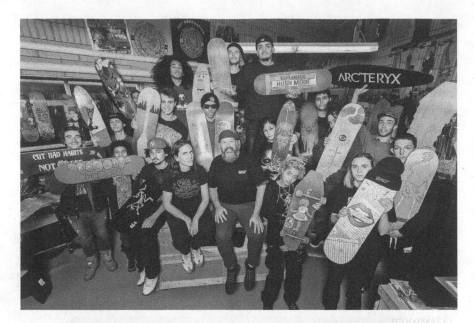

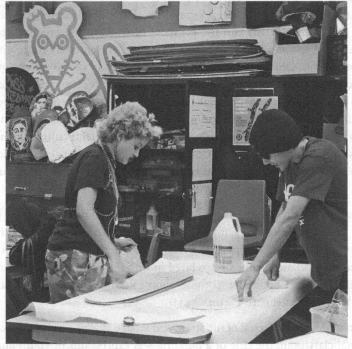

FIGURE 7.5 Oasis Skateboarding Factory space and images.

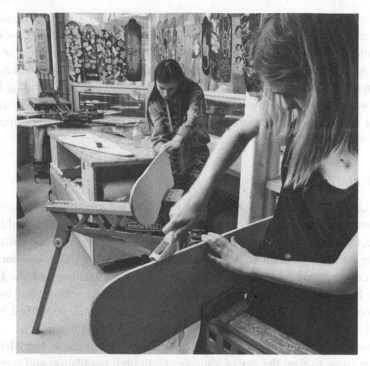

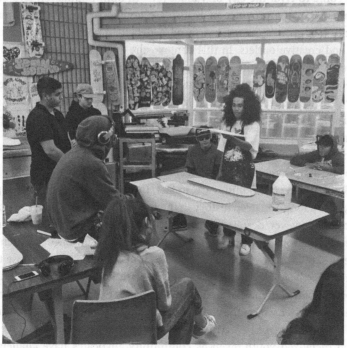

FIGURE 7.5 **Continued**

who have a right to be in public and whose culture of graffiti, electronic music, and street art is not only fit for the times but is also a creative source for future self-realization. In this way, OSF captures the challenge and opportunities for using public spaces in an era dominated by a sociocultural politics of creative economic development and securitization for and in response to youth. Operating in the in-between city, it has become a gathering place for youth from across the region, a place of security where young people can negotiate external relationships and future options.

SOUTH ASIAN ARTS

As in London and Toronto, the 2000s have witnessed growth and transition in Vancouver's youth arts sector. At least seven new organizations launched in this period, extending the spread of the sector beyond the downtown and eastside of the city into suburban areas. At the same time, as funding tightened, not all of these organizations have survived, including Peace It Together and the Purple Thistle Institute. The emergence of YouthSites beyond the downtown and eastside of Vancouver nonetheless marked an important moment, exemplified by the launch of South Asian Arts in Surrey-Newton, British Columbia, in 2005.

Surrey is a large and increasingly complex suburb in the Lower Mainland that has come to rival the city of Vancouver—in both population and economic development—in the province of British Columbia. As in other regional cities, as the city has grown, Surrey has faced a deficit in social and community resources and creative outlets. In this context, the emergence of South Asian Arts in the region highlights the extension of the youth arts sector into historically underserviced suburban cities. Its story also highlights the challenges youth arts have faced in developing spaces of aesthetic diversity and cultural recognition while facing the crosswinds of multicultural cosmopolitanism and powerful global media spectacles.

Surrey is playing an increasingly significant role in the local region. It is also home to one of the largest South Asian enclaves in the world outside of the subcontinent. South Asian communities are, in fact, the largest visibly racialized group in Canada, with a long and deep history in the metropolitan Vancouver region. In recent decades, however, despite increasing public recognition of this history, dominant representations of South Asian youth have focused on delinquency, gang violence, and the threat young Brown (male) bodies are thought to pose to others (Bukhari, 2019). Media coverage of Vancouver-area South Asian youth in the 1990s and 2000s amplified themes of anxiety and threat; at the same time, politicians and journalists have focused on the supposed failures and shortcomings of immigrant families as the source of this crisis. The resulting public discourses have focused blame on racialized youth, even as community advocates have challenged this construction and the negative impact divisive representations of Brown bodies have had for South Asian communities in Canada.

From the outset, South Asian Arts has operated within a mixed economy social enterprise model. It relies on a mixture of fee-for-service programs and targeted state and third-party funding to support training in traditional South Asian dance and music, including Bhangra, Gidha, Kathak, Dhol drumming, and the sitar. It has also produced theater and festivals for professional and amateur South Asian artists. Gurp Sian, a founding director of South Asian Arts, suggested that the purpose of this work was to move South Asian creative expression from the Gurdwara or small private dance schools into more public spaces:

> We wanted to be ourselves, be part of a community that involved arts. Whether it be through teaching [or other work] . . . we wanted to give back to the community. By passing on what . . . we had learned, what was valuable . . . we wanted to pass that on to the next generation. Because . . . when I was younger there was no such thing as Bhangra dance class or Dhol drumming class. (Interview with Gurp Sian, June 15, 2018)

Prior to groups such as South Asian Arts, the South Asian community's involvement in the arts was largely hidden from view and/or subject to racist acts of abuse and disregard. In response, South Asian Arts has worked to claim a space by legitimizing and recognizing South Asian dance, music, and performance as valued forms of cultural expression and professional practice:

> South Asian Canadians are the largest visible minority group in Canada, yet a simple scan of Vancouver's performing arts community suggests that there are very few South Asian theatre professionals currently working in our industry. (Monsoon Festival Program, South Asian Arts)
>
> South Asian Arts aims to balance the lives of adults and children and develop their individuality through the arts. We are committed to artistic excellence through innovation and creativity. It is our mandate to create performance and educational opportunities for professional and amateur artists and build artistic forums and educational opportunities for building knowledge of South Asian cultures via New Projects; New Ideas; New Collaborations. (See https://www.southasianarts.ca)

During their first decade, South Asian Arts programs have been accredited by the local Surrey School Board (for high school credit) and a local university. South Asian Arts has expanded its original programs and developed the Monsoon Performing Arts Festival, an annual celebration hosted in multiple spaces in Surrey and Vancouver featuring workshops, classes, and shows integrating professional and amateur performers. Like other organizations in the region, South Asian Arts has benefited from state and corporate interest in creative economic development and the promotion of cultural diversity. Between 2008 and 2010, for instance, the group partnered with the Organizing Committee of the 2010 Winter Olympics, eventually leading to 17 performances at multiple venues throughout the city during the global festival. Afterwards, it partnered with the National

Hockey League (NHL) and the city's NHL team, the Vancouver Canucks, to celebrate Diwali, the Hindu festival of lights, at the city's stadium arena. South Asian Arts also contributed to the Times of India Film Awards show held in Vancouver in 2013 and has performed at the Canadian music awards show, known as the Junos.

As its work has progressed, the organization has undoubtedly brought considerable visibility to South Asian creative communities and practices. At its home studio in Surrey, for instance, the organization has created a space of belonging and learning beyond the walls of the Gurdwara (Figure 7.6). In a host of other public settings, it has welcomed historically invisible forms of cultural expression into the public gaze. Across its work, it has contested the representation of young Brown bodies as delinquent and dangerous, and it has offered a new cultural calculus to understand South Asian youth. Similar to Paddington Arts' collaboration with Carnival in London, South Asian Arts has leveraged partnerships with mainstream public events, including hockey games, the Olympics, and annual weeklong festivals, as well as institutions such as universities and school classrooms to weave South Asian art practices into spaces of mainstream education, celebration, and engagement. It has challenged how cultural difference is constructed in Canada, by staging Bhangra and other South Asian art forms as part of the fabric of national celebrations and by configuring stages of appearance for South Asian youth, to initiate lines of intersection between South Asian art practices and theater, music, and performance communities in Surrey and across the region. In this way, South Asian Arts has supported symbolic production to counter media panic about South Asian youth. It uses space—in Surrey and beyond—to foster what

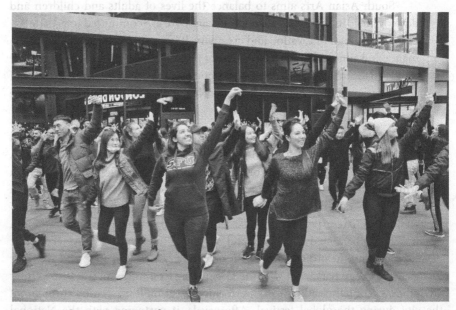

FIGURE 7.6 South Asian Arts performances.

Kathleen Gallagher and colleagues (2020) call "radical hope," a sense that things need not be as they are, that new community relationships with public space are possible, and that forms of celebratory multiculturalism can legitimate meaningful forms of difference in the city.

Conclusion

Making common space for socially disadvantaged young people in cities in the age of neoliberalism has been a key contribution of YouthSites. We recognize that the role of place-making has become more complicated for YouthSites in the wake of the COVID-19 pandemic and the appeal of online forms of gathering, and we return to this tension in Chapter 10, in thinking about the future of the sector. Nonetheless, while responding to the needs of young people increasingly isolated within impoverished, underserviced, in-between regions in cities, YouthSites have themselves emerged as key intermediary organizations, with sometimes deep and abiding relationships with local communities and equally significant dependencies on the state, private funders, and a complex array of partners. They provide young people with a place to stand, to learn, sometimes to eat and make friends, to get tickets for public transit, and to move out into the world. They are a kind of home for participants, a site for "border work," to develop external relationships, negotiate social skills, and imagine possible futures (Christensen & O'Brien, 2003, p. 4).

Paddington Arts has done this work by making a stable community space in an urban region undergoing ferocious forms of change. It has marked the local streets as spaces where young people belong, working with partners such as Carnival to create performative sites as social spaces where young Brown and Black bodies can represent their right to be seen, to claim a place on the streets as their own. In Toronto, OSF has used an urban curriculum infused with the signs, spaces, and art of the city to place young people in the city, within networks and relationships that matter now and possibly in the future. South Asian Arts has likewise created a space of appearance to respond to the needs of racialized youth living in suburban ring regions around Vancouver. Using traditional dance, drumming, and so on, it has marked spaces throughout the region and, in the process, has helped contest how South Asian art and youth are represented and seen in the Canadian imaginary.

Of course, none of this work has been without starts and stops, opportunities and burdens caused by the shifting ground of social provision for youth in a neoliberal era. Since 1990, YouthSites have been dependent on the twists and turns in state financing and policy, and their role in creating youth-specific spaces has paradoxically implicated organizations in the spatial sorting of young people in the city. Amid a broader tendency in the United Kingdom, Canada, the United States, and other countries during the past 30 years to unbundle social services from the state (Graham & Marvin, 2001), YouthSites have developed in cities at a time when traditional modes of state-led corporeal ordering in urban environments have broken down and new, less orderly, structures of infrastructure provision—from roads and sewers to security and social services for young people—have taken the stage. The "unbundled city" (Graham & Marvin, 2001) is a form of neoliberal urbanism that encourages local competition for resources, civic boosterism, and the development of urban cultural brands that "sell" cosmopolitanism and cultural diversity. But these models and their mantras have "largely [been] directed towards mobile, non-local and corporate capital, property developers and high income urban[ites] . . . and professional workers" (Chatterton & Hollands, 2002, p. 97). YouthSites, on the other hand, have been both a salve and a support system in this setting, places for young people to land, to begin, to learn, and to create in cities that have become increasingly fractured, inhospitable, and incapable of addressing the real needs of youth. They have been able to make these gains because of the people who led these organizations over the period, and it is to a discussion of the role of leadership that we now turn.

8

Leaders and Modes of Leadership

Introduction

Unlike the typical institutions of the modern state—schools, hospitals, and even government departments—the organizations we describe in this book were significantly bound up with the personality and profiles of their founders and early leaders. Although we encountered some instances of succession planning and of institutional longevity—a theme we take up in our description of Ovalhouse Theatre in Chapter 9—for the most part, the vision, commitment, cussedness, and faith of key leaders had significant and direct impact on the organization's community. This is both a limitation and a strength. We discussed in the preceding chapters how types of education, modes of learning, forms of performance, and creative practice all flourished precisely in the intersections of inherited tradition, social change, poverty, marginalization, and the drive for social justice; these contradictions gave rise to unique forms of being and learning in the three cities studied (London, Toronto, and Vancouver). Each organization clearly articulated its purpose in the face of wider social opposition as a form of resistance. This organizing "against the grain" gave the organizations distinctive characters, almost personalities, and these, we argue in this chapter, came about as a result of the quality of the individuals who frequently devoted themselves to these organizations. It was the energy and drive of key individuals exploiting opportunities in education, the arts, youth work, and social care, all created in the city because of reforms to neoliberal governance, that gave character and integrity to their daily activities as much as their longer term purpose and function.

This chapter characterizes the energetic and committed people who work with youth arts organizations and also points toward some of the conditions and historical trends that influence the kinds of leadership that last in the youth arts sector. Bianca Baldridge's (2019) study of an after-school program in the northeastern United States points to both the structural and interpersonal elements involved in the design, delivery, and impact of such a program. She highlights how "previous scholarship captures the significance of community-based youth workers in the

YouthSites. Stuart R. Poyntz, Julian Sefton-Green, and Heather Fitzsimmons Frey, Oxford University Press.
© Oxford University Press 2023. DOI: 10.1093/oso/9780197555491.003.0008

lives of marginalized youth" but also notes that "the voices and experiences are absent from broader educational discourse" (p. 208). In her study, the absence is particularly acute in relationship to race and the assumptions about deficit that frequently accompany such provision. Her interest in the voices and experiences of Black members of staff working with their community highlights individual and interpersonal dimensions, and in particular addresses the role that leaders play in defining the ways that organizations work.

There are several factors that shape this chapter: leadership roles, social cultural contexts, and complex discourses. In terms of leadership roles, first, there are the people who identify as the heads of organizations—the artistic directors, executive directors, the heads of school, etc. These people are the main focus of this chapter. The forms of leadership they developed are interesting in their own right but also in the context of contemporary theories of arts management and leadership that animated the sector at the same time. State and welfare-led arts organizations experienced a wave of managerialism and management critique (see Chapter 9) in an attempt to rationalize efficiency, governance, and accountability in sectors in receipt of government funding (see Christie, 2020; Kuppers, 2019).

Second, there are the no less important, but often less visible, facilitators, teachers, and mentors (including people who take on mentoring roles) who have meaningful and sometimes regular direct contact with the young participants. This dimension is especially important for us because the quality of peer relationships in arts-based and community-engaged practice, especially in bringing together people from socially marginalized groupings, seems salient to these organizations' success. It is certainly present in some of the literature about radical arts mentorship (Kuppers, 2019; Shaffeeullah, 2020).

Third, there are significant people working on arts councils, in funding agencies and government, and developing cultural policy who have a direct impact on the way.youth arts are able to be practiced at a given time.

All three of these roles are present as leaders, and some of our interview participants have occupied a variety of these titles. However, for the purposes of this chapter, we focus on the first two.

Individuals, of course, operate within specific historical social, local, and national contexts, including government regulations and trends that shape urban spaces. Because these topics have been explored in depth in Chapter 7, this chapter builds on those and then analyzes leadership in terms of leadership grouping. The first group is made up of the "pioneers" who were instrumental in shaping organizations in the 1970s, 1980s, and 1990s, some of which continue to be part of urban infrastructures today. We are particularly interested in the leaders who made a commitment to the sector and continued to work within it for at least 20 years, often with the same organization. We note two leadership trends that emerged by the 2000s: (a) leaders who are radically committed to the young people with whom they work and who also embrace many neoliberal ways of operating to ensure the success of their organizations; and (b) leaders who explicitly call out the systemic injustices they see propping up the urban arts sector, grudgingly accept the granting structures governments provide, and, very frequently, come from the communities they serve. Both of these kinds of leaders hail from a younger generation and appear to operate differently from those forged in the 1970s' community arts movements.

Leaders work and achieve what they do within wider discourses and framings. The community arts movement of the 1960s–1980s is one such discourse (discussed in Chapter 6); neoliberal economic practices (addressed in Chapter 7; with respect to leadership in urban contexts, see Andris et al., 2021) are another; institutional education and pedagogies (see Chapter 5) are a third. Along with these broad movements are key ideas that influence how we understand the way youth arts leaders carry out the work. These ideas include service-based models moving to assets-based spaces; feminized/feminine leadership and cultures of care; tokenism and self-replicating systemic injustices; and radical mentorship. These four ideas are explored through case studies in this chapter.

The Pioneers

Across the three cities, it was notable how White women most frequently and persistently launched youth arts organizations in the 1970s through to the 1990s. For example, Celia Greenwood launched Weekend Arts College (WAC) Arts (London) in 1978 and retired in 2017; Phyllis Novak started SKETCH (originally called SKETCH Working Arts) (Toronto) in 1990, retiring in 2021; and Elaine Carol began Miscellaneous Productions (Vancouver) in 2000 and remains the Artistic Director. These are all women who have managed and directed youth arts organizations against the odds and then remained in those roles for at least 20 years, and although their stories are different, they shared significant similarities. In addition to being artistically creative, the women working in these organizations seem tireless, impossibly hopeful, deeply caring, and doggedly determined. The working conditions often meant long hours and financial precarity because many of these organizations relied on government project grants each year to be able to continue their programming. Founders' actions and experiences align with observations that link challenges associated with care work and care experts with gender. Mignon Duffy's (2011) sweeping study of American labor and care, for example, argues that "the work of serving the poor and others in need, once defined as charity, became more associated with expert intervention" (p. 42). She identifies care workers such as doctors, nurses, teachers, and social workers, and she claims that what she calls "nurturant care work" is "loosely linked to ideals of White middle-class femininity" and is "one of the prominent stories of the twentieth century" (p. 42).

Because our sample of youth arts organizations was mainly founded by women rather than men, we might speculate that women were willing to work for less money and to make caring for others a significant part of their daily lives. The work is underpaid, underrecognized, and seems to have attracted leaders for whom care is what counts rather than other ways of measuring social value (Care Collective, 2020). Many of the founders started their organizations when they were young—reckless, bold, and entrepreneurial. They frequently noted that they had no idea that their work would be so challenging, or as meaningful. In many ways, these leaders seem like rule-breakers because they do impossible things, but often, the young leaders did not even know that there were rules to be broken in the first place. Only later, when they had begun to achieve some of their goals, did they realize that they needed to become stubborn—to insist on the significance of their work and the value of the young people with whom they worked.

Phyllis Novak, the daughter of White immigrant parents, launched SKETCH in Toronto in 1996. Her involvement with youth arts began in 1990 when the then 25-year-old walked by Evergreen, a drop-in center for youth that is part of the downtown Toronto Yonge Street Mission, and began volunteering there. She was a York Theatre studies graduate and actor, and she suggested that she might start running drama programs and later, visual arts programs. Novak told us that the space was like many drop-in centers in the early 1990s:

> It was a real hot bed of imaginative potential that was just being asked to be re-pressed. . . . I felt like it was also agitating because we were asking people who, in my view, automatically had entrepreneurial spirit and creative ingenuity, we were asking them to sit on their ingenuity and dampen it and just spend the day here and recognize that you just need a holding tank. (Interview with Phyllis Novak, 2017)

Evergreen could not support the arts projects in ways that she wanted because she was interested in more ambitious multi-faith and secular options.

The transition between Evergreen and SKETCH happened through the Drug Project. Working with past Evergreen participant Sue Cohen, and with Loree Lawrence, who already ran a theater program for street-involved youth called the Kensington Youth Theatre and Employment Skills (KYTES), the Drug Project was framed as a unique work experience program, but it was also Toronto's first high-profile street arts festival. Novak relied on her creative networks to support the street art, and she began to raise money through her church community networks to fund arts programming for young people in a space that featured a wide range of supplies and tools. She also discovered that she could connect her newly minted organization SKETCH with a platforming organization called IMAGO Arts that gave SKETCH a charitable number and helped it with accounting until it could do those things for itself. Platforming was a distinctive form of structural organizational growth where new initiatives such as SKETCH could be hosted by organizations that already had physical spaces, accounts, payroll, and so on, and could mentor the new organizations to become independent.

Novak's story is characterized by a kind of mission-driven zeal. As a street community outsider, she brought her education, skills, and personal networks to the development of youth arts. Her experience at Evergreen influenced her early approach to SKETCH. In 2017, she reflected on the language she had used early on in her project:

> I think that that language, in the first 2 years specifically, was still attached to how things worked at Evergreen and how things worked from a service-based model. . . . I remember that being a critical learning curve for me, to reposition things from that to an assets-based space.

Novak's and SKETCH's success stories, although buoyed by Novak's own privilege, were also characterized by personal experience—the power of theater—and with her enthusiasm to get to know the young people and to support their journey to incorporating creative arts into their lives. In 2017, she told us,

> When I was 16 I got involved with theater and it literally, I think, saved my life. So I really feel like I could totally understand that process, but not just on the healing level but on the level of purpose-making and suddenly finding a direction for my life.

In 1996, in her initial notebook and fundraising document, however, she put the focus on the life she had *not* lived, writing the following:

> The constant struggle of meeting basic needs when living on the streets allows little time for the self-discovery, exploration and growth normally associated with adolescence. Street life is tiring, oppressive and keeps youth powerless. The arts relieve the pressures of the street. Youth have a chance to mourn, express and be vulnerable. SKETCH respects the value of imagination and experience in street youth. It is a safe venue for youth to find their voice, healing, hope and direction.

Indeed, she explained later,

> There are many short-term programs where people can get jobs for three or six months, and it's great to have those skills and move forward. But street-life is demanding and youth don't get the time to explore, to build skills, to build a sense of self required to sustain those skills and deal with all their issues. ("Sketching a Portrait," 2000, document in the Sketch Archive)

By 2008, SKETCH was an established, integral part of the Toronto Arts Scene and acknowledged as a winner of the Toronto Mayor's Youth Arts Award. All of the artists we interviewed who had been teenagers in Toronto were familiar with SKETCH, and most had participated in some of the community events, programming, or open studio times. By then, Novak had shepherded the organization through two different locations and would soon be moving into a third—in 2020, she was raising funds to buy a third space free from rent fluctuations and challenging landlords. In less than 10 years, SKETCH had gone from an idea and a group of young people who produced public events such as the Drug Project, without permits, to an organization deeply entrenched in the Toronto youth arts scene.

As an organization leader, Novak was sensitive to the shifting needs of youth who wanted to access SKETCH's resources. In the first space, SKETCH initially attracted street-involved young women and, later, young men. In this venue, the only rules were "do your own dishes" and "sign in," because SKETCH needed such records to justify the grants it received. Everyone could sit and listen to music, and everyone was encouraged to make something. For many young people, the appeal was to have a space where they did not need to be part of a formal program, where they could just *be*. But by the early 2000s, when SKETCH moved to its King Street space, it was popular with young people participating in the punk scene. Novak realized that although SKETCH had approximately 50 active participants each week, many young men would simply come to the SKETCH place to hang out. She explained, "Drop-in spaces, I feel like, are this holdover from . . . post-war when it was men hanging out to get a meal and chat up places and stay warm." Inadvertently, aspects of SKETCH had become the "holding tank" that Novak rejected at Evergreen. When Novak and her team realized that women, especially young women of color, were not participating as much, they applied to Status of Women Canada for funding to get training in gender-based violence and gender-based analysis, in order to learn about why women were not participating. Young women told them that they wanted something constructive that would take them from A to B, which was a message they had not been hearing before. SKETCH changed its operations from an open space studio to one with more structured opportunities. When SKETCH moved into its third space, it also decided to key the doors to the basement studios so that young people had to be formally granted access and could not simply wander in, increasing some participants' sense of safety. More young women, and especially those of color, were recorded as participants.

The structure of the third space, with studios and kitchens in the basement and the administrative offices on the second floor of the building, emphasized some separation between leadership and participants that probably existed less when someone would walk through the lounge. Certainly, while we were conducting interviews through Toronto, Black, Indigenous, and people of color participants would tell us that although they loved SKETCH, it is notable that "as you walk up the stairs, the whiter it gets." Youth arts organizations, in general, have tried to make their programming as accessible as possible to any young people who are experiencing socioeconomic barriers, yet, as the story of young people of color illustrates, different demographics require different provisions to make the space inviting. This is as true now following Black Lives Matter as it was in the early days of many of the organizations we describe. Novak, as a White woman, recognized that SKETCH was not reaching all the young people she thought it should, and she needed to work intentionally to determine why. Her own Whiteness and the privileges associated with that did not mean that she assumed that she understood their lived experiences, or that she imagined she already knew what was best for the young people. Yet, without suggesting that the programming and fundraising Novak does is in any way easy, her Whiteness also probably made it easier for her to move through the Toronto establishment in order to negotiate funding, rent spaces, and promote SKETCH in a positive way to the community. Novak's daily struggles are significantly different from the ones shared by her youth participants.

Novak's leadership story shares many parallels with those of White women youth arts pioneers in London and Vancouver as well. For example, Celia Greenwood, a White drama teacher in London, acknowledged that her class, education, Whiteness, and, as she put it, "social capital" helped her open doors; ensure that her staff were fairly paid; and ensure that she could break down barriers that impeded young people's opportunities, such as racialization, disability, class, and financial means. From the beginning in 1978 when she and a friend successfully approached philanthropist Ed Berman in order to start WAC, as it was then known, to advocating for young people in 2016, Greenwood told us "You need to be a Sisyphus" to continue to insist on pushing the rock up the mountain. "The fucking world's mad, like, why don't they just think like me and give lots of money to [kids, the people who need it]." She also described disheartening stories of young people being refused auditions because of a Black Caribbean accent or because they had not already trained in ballet and also how WAC Arts made it possible for young people to get some of the pre-professional training they needed to move forward in their careers. One thing she knew she needed was a mentor for participants. Although initially it was difficult for her to find Black artists who were confident enough to teach, through WAC she arranged mentorship in teaching skills so that the organization could increase its roster of Black instructors. Another thing they needed was to create structures that allowed for a flexible working environment that could support a range of abilities and health concerns. Greenwood described a talented young woman who had seizures twice a day, who WAC accommodated in its classes. Her deep care for the young people, along with her privileged status as an educated White woman, made it easier—but not easy—for her to advocate for WAC's young participants and the programs WAC offers: "I have been angry all my working life. I haven't got bitter, because it's a joy to work with young people and somehow you make it happen, somehow . . . the anger is to make me fight."

Similarly, Elaine Carol, of Miscellaneous Productions, Vancouver, described the constant fight waged on behalf of the young people. Initially, Miscellaneous Productions had trouble getting charitable status in Canada because it used the word "antiracist" in its mandate, and this was considered politically charged at the time. Carol argued that because the organization's programs explicitly address complex social issues, part of her role in programming is to collaborate with various specialists and artist-activists to effectively address interlocking systems of oppression (bringing forward violence, racisms, and trauma) and to ensure that programming structures are well supported. Carol sees the nuance of her role as a caring leader is for participants to see their own potential to be successful adults and to help young people navigate the challenging world in which they live. As is the case with Novak and Greenwood, the determination, energy, imagination, and selflessness required to do this work cannot be overstated.

The Next Generation

Although initially the majority of youth arts organizations were led by energetic outsiders—external, that is, to the communities they served—in the 2000s leadership began to shift in two main ways. First, some organizations began to be led by young business-driven social entrepreneurs, such as Craig Morrison of Oasis Skateboard Factory (Toronto), Michael Prosserman of Unity Charity (Toronto), and Nii Sackey of Bigga Fish (London). Second, other leaders, who in some significant way share identities or experiences with the demographics of their youth arts organizations—Jason Samilski of CUE, Nikki Shaffeeullah of The Artists Mentoring Youth (AMY) Project, Randell Adjei of RISE Edutainment, Megan Solis of Miscellaneous Productions, and Gurp Sian of South Asian Arts—operated explicitly as radical insiders, aiming to help participants develop strategies and ideas to address systemic injustices, and make visible change from the inside out. Whether their personal story includes previous street involvement or homelessness, lived experience of racism, prejudice related to a non-heteronormative identity, or growing up in the same neighborhoods as the youth they hoped to serve, these young leaders challenged the systemic injustices they saw, accepting government funding while calling out the organizations that fund them. There is definitely a crossover between these two "types," and as demonstrated later, some individuals encompass elements from both strands. In addition, there are obvious points of connections with earlier pioneers, even though there are no data to support findings about the demographic composition of the leaders themselves, given we cannot make any simple characterization of White, middle-class leadership in the past, noting exceptions such as Adonis Huggins of Regent Park Focus Youth Media Centre (Toronto) and Deblekha Guin of Access to Media Education Society (Vancouver). Researchers examining related fields of culturally feminized care work have already begun to study various ways men and racialized people may engage differently with this work (D. Barker, 2012; Puzio & Valshtein, 2022; Wingfield, 2009). They point toward such issues as a racialized "glass elevator/escalator," persistent devaluing of feminized skills, and regular framing of affective care work as a "labor of love." However, for the most part and from what we gleaned from the organizations we studied, this second wave of leaders approached youth arts organizations differently than the earlier pioneers for two reasons. First, the discourses surrounding community service and social change differed from the 1990s onwards. Second, funding opportunities as a result of the move (outlined in Chapters 7 and 9) from welfare provision to enterprise opened up new avenues for growth and development. In other words, we are suggesting that new kinds of leadership style became possible.

When Shaffeeullah spoke in admiration about CUE, she explained how she thought organizations such as these newer ones differed from past organizations:

> I don't necessarily think it's because it's youth-led, though it is. I think it's also because it's led by youth who—like the people who started CUE—are people who were street kids. They really, really understand the community they're serving . . . they have very well informed contexts for doing that work, and have gone through other programs as participants. And I think that goes really far. . . . Where there's difference is that contexts have changed in the ecosystem that has allowed people to be leaders that might have had more barriers to be leaders 20 years ago. So it's not by virtue of being new. It's by virtue of subsequent—it might have been harder in 1990 for something like CUE to form.

There is both an acknowledgment of diverse experiences now leading these community-based organizations and a realization that the shape they took can be explained to a large extent by how they built on the principles and practices established by earlier generations.

ENTERPRISE AND OPPORTUNITY

In Chapter 7, we described Nii Sackey's inspiration to found Bigga Fish in response to a youth center worker's comments regarding police surveillance. His first initiative was an MC/DJ workshop at the youth center, leading to further events. Bigga Fish emerged as a youth-focused events organization, providing performance platforms for young artists, as well as events, marketing, and management training for 14- to 21-year-olds, as we describe in Chapter 9. The organization grew to serve 1,000 young people per workshop, to present workshops in schools for 7 hours a day, and became the largest producer of tours presenting teenaged "creatives."

Although Bigga Fish received funding from a wide range of trusts, foundations, and arts councils, Sackey himself adopted the language and approach of capitalism and business. Rather than calling himself Artistic Director or Producer, Sackey was the CEO. His account of Bigga Fish emphasizes statistics that share big numbers (number of paid staff, number of participants, number of events, and number of financial contributions) rather than a few deep relationships or experiences. In 2004, he won a Clore Leadership award,[1] which he explained in terms of "the numbers—it's all about the numbers . . . [and] about inspirational and visionary leadership." When he talked about engagement, he described the economics of "demand":

> We always used to laugh at the other organizations because they always used to talk about engagement being a problem. Our problem was never engagement,

> or it was engagement in the sense that there was . . . too much kids. And that's
> always been the case that there has always been too much demand. Our moti-
> vation has always been demand and that has been a gift and a challenge for us.

Sackey claimed that the organization was geared toward the "transformation of
young people's lives" beyond the arts—"We're not really a music organization"—
and he also described a 2013 finance scheme he had worked on with the Cabinet
Office that set up 120 businesses, owned by young first-time business owners,
throughout the country. Reminiscent of the Canadian Opportunities for Youth
Fund of the late 1970s[2] that helped so many young people launch their own
businesses, Bigga Fish provided mentorship and training to more than 100 young
people who had been sold loans, "often with very little understanding." Fishterns
(interns), or members of the Street Team, focused on entrepreneurial, branding,
marketing, and budgeting skills while they also earned income and benefits of
their own. Even as government funding sources were drying up in 2017, Sackey
defined his own organization as "innovative" and ready to explore alternative business models to deliver services within the market.

When Bigga Fish became known for events at the Notting Hill Carnival, it
was recruited by the BBC Concert Orchestra, Sirius, and Radio 3 to develop more
mainstream high culture programming and to run a series of events called Urban
Classics. This was the first time Sackey identified racism and a glass ceiling for
Black people in the arts funding system:

> We recognized one of the kind of core truths of the art sector is that the few
> hold the majority of the resources, so, and whereas the masses have crea-
> tivity, so, what I realized during the conception of that project was that the
> orchestras had . . . their performance was very low creativity, very low inno-
> vation, and high levels of resources and quality of execution. However, the
> Grime music scene had high levels of creativity and innovation and low levels
> of resources and lack of access to quality development, so it seemed natural
> to put the two together. And it was supremely successful. And what happened
> was that a year afterwards we went back to them and proposed doing it again,
> making it a regular thing and they said "No" and the year after they came back
> and did it themselves.

Sackey's experience is not, unfortunately, unique. Research contrasting the situation in Scotland and Denmark (Stevenson et al., 2017) demonstrates that part of
the "engagement" problem that Sackey refers to is about how cultural participation is defined in the first place. If popular arts such as the Grime music scene, or
community-engaged arts such as young people DJing, are included in government
statistics, engagement in culture is nearly 90%. However, this is not the kind of
figure collected by national arts councils. An interpretation suggesting 92% of the
UK population do not participate in the arts obscures the fact that citizens are, in
fact, typically engaging in other, nonsubsidized arts activities and may have made

an active choice to use their time and money in another manner. This is the "core truth" Sackey discerned above, so his own version of these statistics was that

> the Arts Council spends 97 percent of its money on orchestras and then . . . especially when you consider 92 percent of an orchestra's audience is White, above the age of 30. And 50 percent is White male and above the age of 50.

This analysis of diversity and participation had implications for Sackey's mode of leadership and possibly his faith in market solutions as he began to lose trust in public funders. He recounted that when the Arts Council of England asked him why he was not applying for funding in the early 2000s, he explained his change of direction in terms of issues to do with race and Urban Classics. He was convinced to apply again on the basis of an increase in grant size, and he worked with the Arts Council from 2002 until 2012. However, in 2012 and 2015, he piloted a children's version of Urban Classics with several orchestras whose engagement levels were, as Sackey stated, shocking, and so he then worked with private donors such as the Andrew Lloyd Weber Foundation to support the project. The Arts Council then cut its funding and, in his words, told him "stay out of classical and stick to Carnival." He was advised that there were "better" people to do the work, even though he had just sold out the Barbican (a large London Arts venue) for an orchestral event:

> What I realized was that I was starting to experience a real glass ceiling . . . and when I began to look into it the Arts Council produced a report in 2015 about the state of the diverse sector and within that they said the music department should get upliftment so even their own reports contradicted their actions. I couldn't understand it.

Sackey believed that the Arts Council had a "quota" of Black organizations to support and once that was filled, it was not interested in relationships with additional organizations. He believed that he and Bigga Fish were being kept in a small, racialized box, denying him resources. Although Bigga Fish continued to win awards and be evaluated highly by the Arts Council, by 2016 it was receiving only 10% of the funding it used to receive from the Arts Council. Sackey accepted these funds "because I've got responsibilities to kids. . . . My only reason to engage with [Arts Council and funders] now is for the benefit of young people. I have a very low level of respect for the sector." Describing it as racist, he said, "Actually there is two sides to the system of what they are doing. One is privilege and one is consequence. So I live with the consequence where someone else lives with the privilege."

Sackey thus refused to give up on a funding system despite its evident contradictions persisting in the marketplace, arguing that young people can and should work the system to their advantage. It is possibly that other younger leaders also operated in less conciliatory terms than their pioneer predecessors. For example, in Toronto, Nikki Shaffeeullah joined the Community Arts Committee, a jury that funds local organizations and that can also advocate for more equitable change within the system. She told us that unlike 5 years ago, the Committee is completely made up of people like her,

> with similar kinds of politics, and they're all Indigenous and racialized. There's a lot of LGBTQ people, and there's a lot of people who had had long-term activist backgrounds in addition to artist backgrounds. . . . I feel excited being in that world because I feel like there's a really strong politic around what community arts can be in terms of equity and access.

The positive attitude is reaching participants as well. Shaffeeullah's practices, as a leader at The AMY Project, demonstrated her commitment to creating changes. After Shaffeeullah was hired as AMY's Artistic Director, she helped expand the organization's mandate from working with "young women" to working with "young women and non-binary youth." She encouraged the staff and board to review their practices, and they realized that there were still barriers they needed to address in terms of how they worked to engage trans-women and so they developed a special poetry program for that demographic. In her article about The AMY Project's radical mentorship policy, Shaffeeullah (2020) writes about the way she, as a leader, believes that the work she does, and the *way* that she structures AMY's work, can disrupt patterns and call attention to, and shift, barriers that some young people experience:

> While all youth deserve education, attention, and access to creative expression, it is youth from certain communities and experiences who face systemic barriers to these things, and that is who we prioritize in our mentorship models. We are interrupting systems of colonialism, racism, classism, transphobia, queerphobia, ableism, misogyny, etc., and our point of intervention is by working to uplift young people living at the intersections of these experiences. (p. 32)

Mentoring and Key Staff

Very few of the founders and leaders we met seemed obsessed with their own charisma or any cult of leadership. Indeed, at an anecdotal level, we were continually impressed by their public-facing doggedness and drive, mixed with their self-effacing service. The leadership was frequently a question of people who had experience working directly with young people, or in education, or as arts practitioners being catapulted into situations in which they had to act as fundraisers, advocates for their organizations, and representatives in frequently very different social arenas from their own. Many of the individuals we met commented on how much of their day jobs were spent with budgets, spreadsheets, and in other forms of practice in which they had to position themselves as learners out of their immediate comfort zone rather than as confident leaders directing others. Indeed, it was a feature of leadership that individuals made do and took responsibility in domains that were often challenging and changeable. None of these organizations could exist without leadership from mentors and the wider staff group who were not the directors but who worked with the young people directly. Many staff members were former participants and were deeply committed to the organization and the community. Some staff were brought in to work with groups or group members as artist-experts for a short-term contract or specifically as mentors.

WAC Arts in London is instructive here. Right from the outset in the late 1970s, one of the founders, Celia Greenwood, recognized that she needed to take responsibility for developing staff who came from the kind of communities students came from. Indeed, some of the very first students returned to work as teachers and key workers at the organization as their professional careers unfolded. Older students were recruited via a system of refunds to act as student assistants. By the early 2000s, there were nearly 200 part-time staff being employed on a yearly basis, of whom approximately 60% were from minority ethnic groups, and virtually all of whom had come through the system as students in the first instance. The culture of care and youth-centered focus thus became habitual—inbuilt into the kinds of relationships students and staff expected. In addition, senior staff who took responsibility for running programs expended considerable energy on pastoral care, following up on absences and taking the time to support individuals in and around the arts-based activities of the organization.

Powerful stories exist throughout the sector. Meg Solis, Assistant Director of Miscellaneous Productions and a choreographer, has a story that resonates with many of the politicized radical insiders who are working to change youth arts organizations and the youth arts scene from within, refusing to accommodate overtures from funders that may not be up to their ethical standards.

Solis started out at Miscellaneous Productions after auditioning as a Grade 12 student. She told us that she was raised in a low-income, working-class, immigrant, Asian family, and all of those factors had previously restricted her potential to access an arts education. Even if those factors had not mattered, she pointed out that there was almost no representation by people of color in theater or the media when she was growing up, so she never imagined a career in the arts was an option for her. "Unfortunately, it is just harder for someone of color and for someone who also presents as a woman," she explained. She added that the opportunities Miscellaneous Productions gave her, the reference letters, and the training and support opened doors for her, such as scholarships, bursaries, and entrance into a theater program, that she believed would never have opened otherwise. After theater school, Solis worked as a freelance choreographer and also as an assistant on Miscellaneous Productions shows. After approximately 2 years, she was hired as the organization's Assistant Director.

Now, as a leader in the organization, she prioritizes mental health and her own emotional availability to the participants. In addition to powerful artistic work, the

thing that differentiates Miscellaneous Productions from other youth arts organizations, in her opinion, is care. Her own experience as a young person finding
community at Miscellaneous Productions and, later, at theater school helped her
aim "to be the best that I can be and offer my best as well," and she is inspired by
"these more artistic folks who were caring enough to establish a sense of community with me . . . that I never would have gotten honestly from home." She argues
that to really benefit from Miscellaneous Productions, participants need to put in
the work, but sometimes

> these kids don't always have the right situation at home, [but] they still can
> gain something from the organization and working with us. Our hope is . . . to
> nurture all the kids who come to us as well as other people who work with us
> as well.

At the time of our interview, Solis was most angry about what she called
"parachute projects . . . they come in, they work with youth, specifically at-
risk youth or Indigenous youth and they do it for like 2 weeks or a month and
they leave. . . . It's really damaging to the community and they don't follow-up."
Whereas Miscellaneous Productions' programming provides appropriate support,
counselors, artists who are familiar with issues, connections to community resources, and more as part of their responsible creation and follow-up processes,
she suggests that some organizations leave kids hanging. Sometimes she believes
the feeling young people have is that they had a really good thing going and now it
is gone. Furthermore, other young people are overwhelmed by the complexity of
the issues raised during a creative project but when the project simply parachutes
in, they are left without continuity of care:

> I feel that we are the only ones [in the area] who can provide all those things
> in terms of the length of a program, the care that goes into it, the accessibility
> of finances but also the . . . the high quality of work we produce in the end.

Care for participants seems to be enshrined in most youth arts organizations, but care for staff is more difficult to come by. Solis has noticed that because
Miscellaneous Productions provides a safe environment, "frustrated youth will
take things out on the artistic director, or some of the staff because we remind
them of other people in their life who should be offering them that care but aren't."
Other leaders talk about similar challenges. Sackey observed that the London
Arts Council does not realize that the work with young people never stops: "My
staff get calls at 1, 2, 5 in the morning from young people." Elaine Carol, Artistic
Director of Miscellaneous Productions, describes herself as nearly burnt out. The
truth is that although many organizations are very intentional about caring for the
young people, the precarity of the work, the uncertainty regarding funding, and
the emotional nature of working with young people who are living in challenging
circumstances all place significant demands on youth arts workers. Although
organizations such as Unity Charity ensure that their staff get benefits and the

organization is understanding about staff mental health needs, leaders rarely believe they can take time off. The relative youthfulness of the staff in these organizations also creates structural problems for long-term career planning, and as a general principle, most workers in the sector rarely have access to the same kind of long-term pensions or pension planning that is more common in more secure care professions.

Leaders and managers at youth arts organizations such as Miscellaneous Productions demonstrate care through what Izatt-White (2011) calls "valuing practices"—actions that demonstrate care in ways that are meaningful to leaders and participants, such as taking abuse from a young person in crisis or taking a late night phone call. As Preston (2013) explains in her work on applied theater practitioners, "Building good, nurturing relationships with young people requires feeling, an investment, sensitivity to individual needs and a genuine show of one's human qualities" (p. 236). She also observes that for self-protection, at times it involves distancing oneself from a crisis so that the facilitator is not too vulnerable to deal with the dilemmas of applied theater work. These dilemmas, Preston argues, are compounded by high-needs participants and market-driven demands by funders or partners that may set up unrealistic expectations along with uncertainty regarding available resources, which can result in a sense of powerlessness. Izatt-White (2011) expands on Hochschild's (1983) well-known concept of "emotional labor," examining managers in colleges, differentiating between emotional skills (which help leaders read emotions and manage their own and the emotions of others), and emotional displays (which include performed friendliness and service with a smile or, in the case of leaders, valuing practices that ensure that staff believe they and their work are valued) (Izatt-White, 2011, p. 10). While paying attention to how emotional labor skills can be leadership tools rather than follower requirements, her sample nevertheless focuses on the mundane leadership situations. Clearly, young participants at Miscellaneous Productions feel valued because the leaders engage in valuing practices that are meaningful to the young people, such as answering phone calls from them in the middle of the night.

In response to the care work mentorship in youth arts organizations demands, The AMY Project set up a structure for what Shaffeeullah (2020) calls "radical mentorship," which, for her, first and foremost is a pathway to equity. One of the key features of The AMY Project is that it pairs young participants with a mentor. Shaffeeullah writes, "We have experienced, learned, and observed that artists seeking mentorship look for it from those whom they feel connection to for reasons beyond disciplinary commonalities; mentorship relationships are often enriched when the mentor and the mentee share experiences, identities" (p. 32). In practice, the Director and General Manager at The AMY Project ask the young person what they are looking for, in order to avoid making assumptions about what would be meaningful in the young person's life. Then AMY seeks out mentors to pair with young participants. Mentors agree to meet with young people 10 times for 10 hours in total. They are encouraged to place barriers around their time but also to share their professional work (e.g., inviting the mentee to their rehearsals or to attend a show together).

What makes the program radical is that (a) the mentees get to request the kind of person they want to be mentored by and (b) AMY recognizes and aims to reduce the burden of being a mentor. In particular, the manifesto Shaffeeullah has written for The AMY Project and for others notes, "because of systemic barriers, many groups are underrepresented in the professional arts industry. . . . This means that professional artists from these communities are often doing more mentorship and caretaking than their counterparts. It's an inequitable distribution of emotional labor" (2020, p. 32). Furthermore, because potential mentors, through lived experience, know how challenging it can be, due to systemic barriers, to achieve what they have achieved in their careers, they recognize the need young people have, and it can be very difficult to say "no." So AMY works to make saying "yes" less of a burden: It provides opportunities for free shared meals, finds tickets to productions, creates spaces for creative collaboration between mentor and mentee, and pays a fee for the mentor's time. It also provides mentorship training that includes discussions on setting boundaries between the mentor and mentee, communication strategies, a compiled list of "how to be a great mentor" strategies from past participants, and thought-provoking and critical discussions about resources if there are concerns about the young person's safety. In addition, to support the care work mentors offer, The AMY Project advocates to challenge complacent thinking and encourage "popular understanding of mentorship as an incredibly valuable contribution to the [arts] industry, and a high-status role, in a wider patriarchal society where teachers, nurses, social workers, and other caretaking roles are invisibilized and seen as low-status" (Shaffeeullah, 2020, p. 32).

Conclusion

The trajectory of an organization gives some insight into the power and influence of its leaders and, indeed, how leadership is manifested, but it is difficult for us to capture the host of daily interactions and the ways that relationships develop and unfold over time. Given that all of these organizations had flat structures so that the leaders were significantly involved in day-to-day activities, spending time with young people, and, if needed, ferrying them to the hospital or sitting down and having a meal with them, leadership clearly means much more than simply determining policy direction and smooth bureaucratic functioning. The fact that these organizations both worked directly with young people and also addressed, at times quite significantly, high-status funders, philanthropists, and other more established audiences also meant that the leaders had to be comfortable moving between different types of social interaction, often in a short interval of time.

This chapter has tried to give a flavor of an extraordinary range of people, mainly women, all of whom exhibited similar personal qualities, flair, initiative, care, and imagination. We have tried to show how some of these interpersonal and relational attributes sit within changing cultural and social contexts and are themselves often at the cutting edge of complex discourses relating to social oppression, racism, and other forms of highly sensitive and fraught moments, where groups and communities were often brought into conflict with the mainstream. A considerable quality of "fight" energized much leadership style—a sense of being able to stand up for others and to turn rhetoric into practical, tangible differences in the life opportunities of the young people these organizations served. This is a notable contradistinction to the discipline of arts management developing over the period that saw the emergence of a number of qualifications and university-based courses in the field and that emphasized forms of managerialism we discuss in Chapter 9 that have generically spread across public sector organizations since 1990.

We have noted in particular how forms of radical political position that directly refuted systemic injustice, especially around racial conflict in the three cities, infused leadership styles, helping make these organizations spaces for oppressed or marginalized communities to come together, unite, and celebrate their strengths. This also means noting the attritional effects of sustaining these organizations in the face of what often appeared to be a lack of support and a rejection of values. Leadership is very much simply not giving up as much as it involves ways of turning care into constructive interventions and relationships into concrete ways to develop futures. This is a good jumping off point to reflect on what these organizations have achieved over time in the three cities. It may well be that the era of neoliberalism that started in the 1980s, and which so changed the principles and practices of the social democratic welfare state, is itself beginning to take on new forms and structures. It also may well be that the forms of community arts—based organization that so sustained young people's lives during this period are coming to an end. As we reflect on what these forms of organization achieved during the past 30 years, we also need to face up to whether they represent ongoing, viable moments of institutionalization, in both an increasingly digitalized social life and a precarious labor market.

9

The Paradox of Enterprise

GOVERNANCE, MARKETS, AND SOCIAL GOOD

Introduction

As outlined in Chapter 1, the organizations we studied consolidated into what we have termed the "non-formal learning sector" in the wider political context of neoliberal reform of the welfare state. We argue in this chapter that this context enabled growth and enterprise supporting visions of service, community, education, and the arts, as we have shown in Chapters 5–8. The entrepreneurial imagination of key individuals coming out of social movements, as described in Chapter 8, was given space and opportunity by the move from welfare provision by the state to services provided by social enterprises. However, we also show, through the ways that the organizations metamorphosed in their local contexts, how forms of neoliberal governance determined some of the ways the organizations shaped themselves to appear fit and competitive in the changing marketplaces of the enterprise state.

In Chapters 5 and 6, we described how the youth arts sector operates on the boundaries between a series of relationships comprising state and civil society: formal and non-formal education, arts and social service, and popular culture and formal aesthetic traditions. Institutions are typically publicly funded and yet, even here, they blur divisions between domains that have traditionally been distinct. They are not generally under the remit of any one state department, and they must negotiate support across state departments, including education, arts and culture, health, employment and jobs training, and so on. Organizations are also commonly supported by philanthropic foundations and sometimes offer fee-for-service programs in the marketplace. The Appendix shows both the huge range in funding and the diversity of funding sources for all of the organizations. This "mixed economy" is quite different from the more single-issue, single-sector-funded kind of governance arrangement that frequently characterized these organizations prior to the 1990s. At that time, many of the organizations were

YouthSites. Stuart R. Poyntz, Julian Sefton-Green, and Heather Fitzsimmons Frey, Oxford University Press.
© Oxford University Press 2023. DOI: 10.1093/oso/9780197555491.003.0009

established as projects or initiatives funded by a single source—frequently local government—and often the people who eventually ran the organizations were direct employees of a local authority or other state welfare provision. These embryonic organizations might have applied to one or two charities or local foundations for support for additional projects, such as the way that Weekend Arts College (now WAC Arts) was originally funded by the London Arts Board (now part of Arts Council England) but raised additional funds from both a charity and the local London Borough of Camden to offer classes during the summer holidays for young people with learning difficulties.

Over the period we studied, we can trace the evolution of a range of institutional forms, including stand-alone charitable and/or nonprofit organizations, private companies limited by guarantee (with charitable status), platformed organizations (projects that have been "grown" as part of larger community-based infrastructure organizations), and extension programs embedded in larger cultural institutions. This is captured in the Appendix. Further back in the past, we can trace the history of social service work in and through the arts to provisions offered by religious and labor groups prior to World War II. London's Ovalhouse Theatre was founded as a community center—largely a club for boys—in the 1930s by Christ Church (Oxford) United Clubs, and in Toronto and Vancouver, early settlement houses performed related roles.

We argue here that the change witnessed since 1990 came about as a result of a particular kind of struggle over the growth of funding regimes that emerged in response to the privatization of welfare funding and the implementation of forms of new public management galvanized ultimately by the energies of social enterprise. We describe the difficulties organizations had in morphing into fully fledged businesses and, in particular, the stresses that emerged between organizations forced to diversify and become accountable to different control mechanisms, individuals and projects required to comply with different kinds of scrutiny and outcome measures, and the simple economics of capturing market share and securing longevity and property within increasingly hostile cities. We suggest that these tensions are best understood as a form of neoliberal governance, but to begin here, we follow revenue and material support, showing how these developments shaped organization structures and program delivery over time.

The Pressures of Public Scrutiny, Youth Brands, and the London Property Market: Ovalhouse and Roundhouse

Located in Brixton in the south of London (a traditionally Afro-Caribbean–settled neighborhood), Ovalhouse is a medium-sized youth arts center with a budget in 2015 of £1,029,957 and a long and outsized reputation as a space for promoting experimental, radical, and overlooked arts in the city. It is credited with providing early support for groundbreaking companies in the 1970s (e.g., Foco Novo, Bread and Puppet Theatre in the United States, and the Pip Simmons Theatre Group), and like other groups in our sector, it has staked some of its reputation on its role in launching the careers of musicians, writers, and directors, including Athol Fugard, Pierce Brosnan, Gary Oldman, and Mike Figgis (Woddis, 2007).

In the 1960s, the Ovalhouse became a youth arts center, when Peter Oliver, a mostly unheralded leader of British alternative theater and founder of London's fringe theater, turned a fairly staid youth club into one of London's most exciting experimental arts centers. Oliver is attributed with guiding "a whole new generation and artistic movement into life" with work that was "playful, political, rigorous, international and totally uncompromising" (Woddis, 2007). If Oliver's spirit and drive were essential to the rise of youth arts at Ovalhouse, revenue came from a mix of national arts money, municipal and provincial education/youth services funding, and third sector donations. These included support from the Inner London Education Authority (ILEA), the local Lambeth Amenity Services, the Peter Minet Trust, and the Arts Council of Great Britain (now Arts Council England) (Ovalhouse annual report, 1978).

The ILEA funded classes, workshops, and community youth work programs by supporting the employment of "two full-time youth and community workers and a total of twenty part time youth workers and tutors" (Ovalhouse annual report, 1984). Meanwhile, the Arts Council of Great Britain provided subsidies for "the wages of three full time theatre workers" and the London Borough of Lambeth provided "financial back-up for those salaries which [were] not 100% funded by [Ovalhouse's] main grants . . . together with a small contribution to [their] running costs" (Ovalhouse annual report, 1984). If the 1970s and 1980s were about experimentation, the late 1980s were "a very uncertain time for places . . . like us, [that] rely on grants from statutory bodies" (Ovalhouse annual report, 1984). A victim of "the gradual weaning down of resources . . . [and support] in Inner London and all over the country" (Ovalhouse annual report, 1984), Ovalhouse felt the effects of the Thatcher government's dissolution of ILEA and other granting bodies. By the early 1990s, the organization was faced with a "dramatically reduced budget" (Ovalhouse annual report, 1994). It reached its low point in 1995 when revenue amounted to £742,556 (in 2015 adjusted figures).

With fewer resources to draw on, the diversity of programming at Ovalhouse became unsustainable, and it was forced to specialize and concentrate on professional training and training for progression routes into theater. Deborah Bestwick, the longtime Artistic Director of Ovalhouse (1995–2020), explains the transition:

> We had lots of classes and workshops . . . you know, tap dancing classes and all sorts of stuff. But funding was really disappearing. Ovalhouse as a young people's center had always had a massive grant from the Inner London

Education Authority which was going. . . . So I actually made an initially un-popular decision which was to . . . introduce a theater policy of support for early career artists and new artists. . . . And by making our focus nurturing artists in the professional field, professionally and artistically, we would create better pathways for our young people who wanted to do the same thing and we would look seriously at a rigorous pathway for supporting young people coming into the arts who wouldn't necessarily have the chance to go through the established academic routes and wouldn't have those networks, etc. (Interview with Deborah Bestwick, 2018)

The move to focus on dedicated pathways into the arts for youth was a response to changes in funding, but it also marked a shift toward more direct alignment between Ovalhouse's work and the development of labor markets, a pattern that became increasingly common across the sector in the 2000s. As funding for a mix-ture of training classes became "unsustainable," Ovalhouse's turn to focus more exclusively on youth theater, project-based theater work with specific groups, and ongoing mentorship and training schemes also underlined the emergence of a new pattern of alignment between youth arts and the work of social integration in the 2000s (interview with Deborah Bestwick, 2018; Ovalhouse annual report, 2017). In 2005, following "a significant upgrade" in funding from the Arts Council England (ACE), ACE became Ovalhouse's most significant source of income, representing 41% of its total revenues (£1,050,820 in 2015 adjusted figures) [Christ Church (Oxford) United Clubs, 2005; interview with Deborah Bestwick, 2018]. Total income for that year marked the high point in Ovalhouse's income for youth arts during the past three decades.

This narrative of program reform and efficiency and of a restructure to take advantage of changing funding regimes is not just a story of market responsiveness; it is also a response to perilous financial circumstances that were more exposed to public scrutiny through changes to the publication and control of the financial accounts of companies granted charitable status in the United Kingdom. The de-velopment of the Statement of Recommended Practice (SORP) and the associated, specific requirements for "Accounting and Reporting by Charities" (Hyndman & McMahon, 2010) facilitated this change.

Key to the SORP was the implementation of stronger auditing oversight of the charities sector, along with requirements that charities improve their perfor-mance indicators to allow the state, foundations, and other decision-makers to assess charities "in terms of output and efficiency" (Hyndman & McMahon, 2010, p. 458), while strengthening a "focus on achievements against objectives, organi-zational impact and future strategy, and improved methods for apportioning cost and expenditure to allow more meaningful comparison to be made" (Cabinet Office, 2002, para. 6.12). The SORP facilitated rigorous arm's-length oversight of social services groups through a new reporting regime designed to facilitate trans-parency and the means for comparison across organizations. The integration of the SORP also brought with it a new mandate geared toward professionalism and public relations, dynamics that transformed youth arts from a burgeoning movement of community organizations in the 1980s and 1990s to a sector made up of increasingly specialized organizations capable of negotiating their value with the state and secondary and tertiary funders, while working in the service of community.

In Ovalhouse's 1995 and 2005 annual reports, it is possible to see how these changes, marked by the move to the SORP coincided with an increasing professionalization of the organization at the level of board governance and in the manner of reporting and oversight. The transformation in board membership between 1995 and 2005, for instance, is striking in the sense that the earlier period marked the end of the directorships of 50% of the board (by 1999). By 2005, the board of trustees was nearly 20% smaller and included a media regulator (Eve Salomon) and an auditor (Merle Campbell) among other professionals in its ranks. Reporting by the organization also changed. The 2005 annual report is nearly three times the length of the 1995 annual report, and in line with the SORP's expectations, it includes a much more detailed accounting of organizational structure and fundraising; an extensive "Review of Activities and Future Developments," which did not exist in the 1995 annual report; and a much more detailed accounting of Ovalhouse's financial activities.

In Chapter 7, we described the complex relationship between these organizations and the way they acted as new kinds of space for youth in the city. As we noted, in large cities, property value is a crucial driver of change. Ovalhouse has always existed around a building, the first of which was constructed in 1937, but by 2015 Ovalhouse came to rely on rental income from their buildings, including rent "for music gigs and events, and from the linked bar, catering and box office services." In the mid-2010s, a new Ovalhouse was built—rebranded as Brixton House—which opened in 2021. As Deborah Bestwick clarified, Ovalhouse's new building has had as much to do with creating new revenue lines as it did with the creation of a new space for youth arts:

> We can't make Ovalhouse survive for the next couple of decades on this site because statutory funding through the Arts Council won't go up and we can't make ourselves hostage to fortune . . . by remaining so dependent on Arts Council funding. . . . We're going to have seven rehearsal studios to rent out. (Interview with Deborah Bestwick, 2018)

The lure of new space is compelling, and the apparent obviousness of Bestwick's reference to the risks of overreliance on public funds reminds us of how naturalized austerity thinking has become. Social provision continues to be advanced as a primary objective, but this is now routed through a new and potent mix of conditions that emphasize market exchange, competition, professionalization, and public relations—a very different set of conditions and performance markers than were present in an earlier era.

THE ENTERPRISE OF YOUTH ARTS

Where Ovalhouse tells one story about changes in governance in the sector over the past three decades, the Roundhouse presents a related tale of change. The Roundhouse is a huge, hulking, brick building—originally designed as a railway turntable—sitting at one end of Camden Town's flea market. Now one of the most expensive property areas in the capital, the area has a reputation for trendy shopping, youth-oriented Bohemia, and a dynamic cultural and arts street life. The building itself however, has had a fraught history as an arts venue aspiring to be the hub of the neighborhood.

The first arts center at the Roundhouse was set up in the early 1960s, led initially by playwright Arnold Wesker and, later, by theater producer Thelma Holt. By the late 1980s, support for the Roundhouse had evaporated and the building became derelict. Schemes to develop a Black arts center on site petered out in the early 1990s, and the moribund state of the Roundhouse did not change until 1996 when the intervention of toy manufacturer, Torquil Norman, and support from the New Labour government through National Lottery funds underwrote its resurgence as a state-of-the-art performance space and creative center for young people (interview with Marcus Davey, CEO of Roundhouse, 2018). Torquil Norman eventually invested £7 million in the Roundhouse and set about "lobbying everyone from the Prime Minister and Lord Chancellor down" for support (Morrison, 2006).

The change in funding and support for the Roundhouse was fueled by several factors that marked a strategic shift in the provision of training in the cultural sector, including: (a) the decline of arts revenue funding by the state and the need to operate in a mixed service economy; (b) an emphasis on social value—especially in respect of serving London's young Black communities—needing to be explicit in organizations' activities; and (c) the effects of gentrification on the previously rundown inner city and the exponential growth of the London property market. New Labour's cultural and urban policies shaped and reflected these shifts, and the Roundhouse, responded to the state's invitation. Under the New Labour government, "youth culture was being championed and it was exciting," and during the mid-2000s, New Labour ministers, including the Secretaries of State for Culture, Media and Sport, Chris Smith (1997–2001) and, later, Tessa Jowell (2001–2007), made a point of "coming round" to youth art centers (interview with Marcus Davey, 2018), highlighting the role arts organizations were seen to have as sites of investment and provision for youth.

The arts center (to be distinguished from its role as a public venue) at the Roundhouse officially opened in 2005 with support from philanthropists, National Lottery funds, the Camden Council, and third sector money, offering a wide range of programming in music, the performing arts, the circus arts, and digital media. It promoted its "celebrated Bloomberg Broadcast Programme," training young people in camera operation, direction, and live editing (Roundhouse annual report, 2008), as well as training for an "in-house, youth-powered radio station"

(Roundhouse annual report, 2015). As discussed in Chapters 5–7, many organizations developed relationships with local schools, whereas others, including Roundhouse, made forays into further or higher education, "working in partnership with City University to host the first year of their Events Management foundation degree course" (Roundhouse annual report, 2008). Renewed interest in youth arts thus produced opportunity, but it also produced a new regime of governance (a term we return to later) that wed the sector more directly with the state, labor markets, and targeted educational outcomes. Changes in financing and management in the sector were crucial to this turn.

Roundhouse's 2005 annual report lists the board of trustees, as well as the organization's executive team, along with an extensive breakdown of Roundhouse's objectives and activities, plans for future periods, details on the structures of governance, and a Trustees' Responsibility Statement that marks out what board directors agreed to do, in accepting their positions. By 2007–2008, the annual report highlighted the development of a new Roundhouse Youth Advisory Board, reflecting the SORP's recommendation that those impacted by organizations have a role in their governance. The 2008 annual report also listed the organization's ambassadors (including Sir Bob Geldof, Dame Helen Mirren, Ewan McGregor, and Alan Rickman, among others), a Major Projects Board, and a list of major supporters of projects and core costs. Its design is new, with attention to visual effects showcasing programs, events, and, most important, the participants. In this way, the 2007–2008 annual report reads like a public relations document, one that marks the Roundhouse's professional and celebrity networks, while highlighting key benchmarks for program success and trumpeting how youth arts leads to jobs and the prospect of higher education.

The 2000s thus marked a period of integration and restructuring. Compared to earlier generations, governance in the sector increasingly came to reflect corporate sensibilities, while financing and support were increasingly tied to programs leading to youth participation in the creative industries and progression into higher education as opposed to an older language of "the Arts" or to more community-centered concerns (see Chapter 6). The language and appeal of targeted work with "the hardest to reach" continued, but the representation and orientation of this work shifted: "The Roundhouse" as reflected in a pull-out quote from the 2007-2008 report, became "a breeding ground for the next generation of creative talent." In the same document, the organization's mission statement states that Roundhouse aims "to provide an environment and facilities where young people can engage with artists, industry professionals and their peers to further creative aspirations, vocational opportunities and personal development" (Roundhouse annual report, 2008, p. 5). Finding one's voice, supporting personal development, and opening up prospects for future employment were all important and had, in fact, become the new calling cards of a sector increasingly charged with the work of social provision under a burgeoning regime of market-oriented governance.

Whereas the 2000s were a period of transition and restructuring, by the 2010s, the growing youth arts sector was again threatened by cuts. In the aftermath of the global financial crisis of 2008 and 2009, Davey and others were lamenting that changes in education policy following the demise of New Labour and the rise of a new Conservative government in the United Kingdom had led to funding shortfalls and a new and more complex environment for youth arts organizations. In this context, intensive forms of regulation and oversight continued, while a new challenge emerged.

Between 2008 and 2015, Roundhouse's public funding declined measurably as a consequence of government cuts to the budgets of the Department of Culture, Media and Sport (–24%) and to ACE (–36%) between 2010 and 2014. Before "the cuts," says Davey, Roundhouse received approximately £1,400,000 from ACE, but in the aftermath that figure was reduced by a third to £950,000 by 2018. In other words, by 2015, "for every £1 of public subsidy received" by Roundhouse, it "generated nearly £10 in private revenue" (Roundhouse annual report, 2015).

The reality of this logic settled in forcefully, and by the mid-2010s, in response to the desocialization of revenue, Roundhouse moved to diversify its income. By 2015, its roster of support included funding from ACE, Youth Music, Paul Hamlyn Trust, Atkin Charitable Foundation, Esmée Fairbairn Foundation, Andrew Lloyd Webber Foundation, The Monument Trust, The W. Garfield Weston Foundation, John Lyon's Charity, Amy Winehouse Foundation, and the Rachel Charitable Trust; corporate donors included the Bloomberg Industry Group, Universal Music Group, and ASOS Design; alongside private donations and an additional 26 private partners. By comparison, in 2005, Roundhouse's primary money came from five sources: ACE, Camden Local Area Council, Paul Hamlyn Trust, The Nominet Trust, and the Department of Education. Davey notes that by 2015, the organization's income from public money had declined to 8% of the overall budget, with the remainder of funds coming from trusts, foundations, donations, fee-for-service activities, and commercial ventures (Roundhouse annual report, 2015).

Social Enterprises and Youth-Led Organizations

Where the consolidation of a new regime of governance focusing on the social and property marketplace impacted older youth arts organizations, it also guided the emergence of newer youth arts groups. Unity Charity in Toronto is an instructive example. In 2003, founder Michael Prosserman was invited to create a business plan for his senior entrepreneurship class that would raise money for charity. Prosserman's initial entrepreneurship venture raised money to combat youth violence, and following a stint at York University, where plans were developed, Prosserman and his team branded the project Unity Charity and the organization was launched as a registered nonprofit in 2007.

From the outset, Unity Charity was operated on a mixed-economy, social enterprise model, with fee-for-service work combined with sponsorship, project-based grant funding, and donations to support a hip-hop–infused program that includes training in urban art/graffiti, spoken word, various styles of dance, break-dancing, emceeing, beatboxing, and DJing. In Canada, social enterprises are listed as nonprofit (charitable) limited companies that rely on entrepreneurial activity to address a social cause or mission. Compared to more traditional nonprofits, social enterprises tend to sell services or products, and most often they present themselves as businesses built around a social mission.

By 2015, Unity had grown to offer various strands of programming for "youth living in priority/high risk communities" in Toronto (Unity Charity annual report, 2014, p. 8), with extension and allied programs in smaller Canadian cities, including Calgary and Halifax. A key aim of each program is to promote mental health and the overall well-being of participants through in-school and after-school programs (Unity Inspire programs and the Unity Festival); training programs (Unity Engage); and concerts, panel discussions, and occasional keynote talks. In 2015, Unity offered 23 weekly programs that reached more than 40,000 youth throughout Canada. The Unity Festival kicked off in 2010, and by 2015, it had become a nationwide urban arts gathering aiming to nurture youth identity development while empowering young people with confidence and life skills to manage stress and improve mental well-being (Unity Charity annual report, 2014, p. 9).

Unity is managed by an executive team that, according to the 2015 annual report, works with a board of directors, a Strategic Partnerships Committee, a small Governance Committee, a Festival Working Group, a Finance Committee, and a Programs and Evaluation Committee. Young people, including former program participants, are integrated into the leadership structure at most levels. Black, Indigenous, and people of color (BIPOC) make up more than 50% of the staff leadership group, are a presence on the board, and are, otherwise, highly visible throughout the annual reports. Much like the later reports from Roundhouse, Unity's 2013, 2014, and 2015 annual reports are decidedly visual. They read like public relations documents, complete with visual information graphics showing financial statements; future focus; special events and funders; images of staff, special project participants, and versions of the Unity brand; and images marking major organizational milestones. Both the 2014 and 2015 annual reports include extensive listings and logos of sponsors as well as two pages dedicated to recognizing various levels of donors.

Beyond design issues, what stands out most about the governance structure at Unity is the degree to which membership is divided between largely BIPOC youth and representatives from corporate and other professional worlds. Among the board of directors in 2015, 9 out of 11 members came from the corporate sector, with most hailing from finance and investment. The role and place of corporate imagery, corporate representation, and corporate design in the 2014 and 2015 annual reports highlight the degree to which the mandate on social inclusion and social uplift at Unity is rooted in the mechanisms of market rationalization and corporate social service. Unity's financing tells a similar story.

In 2015, total revenues were CA$1,213,995: 48% of funds came from corporations and sponsorships; 34% from program fees and product and event sales; 4% from private foundations; and 5.5% from holdover revenues. The remaining 8.5% came from government funding. By 2015, Unity thus represented an increasingly dominant model in this sector: an organization driven by a social mandate that is governed by a model of entrepreneurial development, corporate partnership, and social innovation. The early charismatic leadership of founding director, Michael Prosserman, remains a strong presence, and the work of social provision through the arts is largely conceived as a market-centered practice that aims to inspire healthy identities and highly visible youth voices.

RACE AS ENTERPRISE

The visibility of BIPOC youth in Unity's (and Roundhouse's) public profile is significant on a number of levels. Despite the fact that funding for many organizations was both explicitly and implicitly directed toward minority ethnic youth, most organizations were not led by people of color. We return to this issue in Chapter 10. Here, we note how the presentation of racial difference plays a role as both a "problem" and a "solution": justifying public expenditure in the first place; validating investment in the inner city; and commodifying the very processes of marginalization that act as the foundations of deep-seated injustice, poverty, and oppression in the first place. In Chapter 6, we explored the multifaceted nature of "Black arts," drawing particular attention to a series of tensions: the promulgation of high culture to communities denied access, the maintenance and monetization of "othered" novelties within the cultural marketplace, and attempts to redress discrimination and exclusion of the racialized urban cultural workforce. All of these tensions are exemplified through the trajectory of the London-based organization Bigga Fish.

As Anne McClintock (1995) reminds us, the racialization of cultural production has a long history in the West, linked to the legacies of imperialism and capitalism and the colonization of the "Other" for profit. Drawing on the work of Nisha Kapoor (2013), Anamik Saha (2018) argues that in recent decades, "neoliberalism has ushered in a new racial moment, where 'race has become increasingly de-politicized as the state has more vehemently attempted to separate it from structure'" (p. 63). The result is the rise of what Goldberg (2009, 2012) calls "racial neoliberalism," a mode of racial governance in which "Otherness" is produced through the aestheticization of commodities and the "contestation of race, power and ideology" in the service of markets and commodity networks (Baldridge, 2019, p. 8). Baldridge's (2019) study, *Reclaiming Community: Race and the Uncertain Future of Youth Work*, argues that "the pernicious racialized market-based reforms to public education" in the United States and other jurisdictions have been especially harmful for community-based programs (p. 13). Bigga Fish's history is tied to these tensions.

Bigga Fish launched in 2001 as a DJ training program offering fee-for-service workshops in schools. Early ancillary funding was provided through partnerships with larger social services groups such as the Cross River Partnership in London, as well as funds for urban regeneration and some initial small arts grants. The organization grew quickly, and by 2005 it had 18 full-time staff. In a 2018 interview, Nii Sackey of Bigga Fish stated, "We were providing talent workshops, young people from schools were performing, and then we were running workshops in organizing and producing events." Under Sackey's direction, by 2008 Bigga Fish became the largest producer and promoter of teenage music events in the United Kingdom, hosting national tours and playing a key role in the emergence of new musical genres, including Grime (a British variant of hip-hop). While embedded in urban youth culture, Bigga Fish built links with institutions focused on culture-based entrepreneurship and regeneration, and it established collaborations with mainstream arts organizations, including the BBC and the Mayor's Cultural Leadership Board. Throughout its history, Bigga Fish has hosted shows at the Hackney Empire club, contributed to the 2012 Summer Olympics Festival, and has been a regular contributor to the Notting Hill Carnival. The organization is currently housed in a workspace in a luxury innovation and creativity hub in the heart of London's East End technology cluster.

Operationally, Bigga Fish functions as a social enterprise youth talent recruitment agency, in which entrepreneurial-led growth and brand development are used to support youth voices and the development of "transferable lifelong skills" that young people can "take on into their chosen career" (Bigga Fish website, October 2018). As such, Bigga Fish is an interesting example of a social service and innovation project simultaneously exploiting Blackness and creating opportunities for Black youth as "subject[s] whose racial difference is the source of brand value celebrated and marketed as diversity" (Saha, 2018, p. 65).

Within this work, the celebration of cultural difference is both constructive and pernicious. It drives the development of new youth voices and expressions, and yet, as Stuart Hall (2000) noted about "corporate multiculturalism," the celebration of cultural difference as a mechanism for brand development and the marketing of diversity risks reducing the struggle over race to the affirmation of a market calculus as the means for reconciling social relations. The tensions associated with this position are very much a part of the contradictory space Bigga Fish has occupied in the youth arts sector. While recognized for promoting and marketing the sounds and representations of Black minority ethnic youth in the United Kingdom, at the same time, Bigga Fish has been impaired by residual conditions that shape the racialized production of culture in the United Kingdom.

Signs of difficulties were part of the founding of the organization. Sackey notes that Bigga Fish was born from a moment of political injustice:

So basically . . . I was working for a pop group, just as an office . . . gofer . . . and I got talking to a youth worker outside who said "Oh you will never guess what—the police came by today and said they wanted to set up a surveillance operation on top of the youth center to catch some local young people." And it just struck me as being really uncomfortable and just kind of wrong really. I didn't think it was the right way to deal with young people. . . . What came out of that was a sense of . . . wanting to do something about it. (Interview with Nii Sackey, 2018)

Bigga Fish's financing has always included a combination of corporate sponsorship and fee-for-service, with some government-funded public support. Part of its appeal to larger industry partners has been its ability as a grassroots talent and events management development vehicle to feed larger arts organizations and the music industry with workers and innovation (e.g., Grime). In this role, Bigga Fish has a record of engaging large numbers of young people and particularly Black and minority ethnic youth and young people considered "at risk" by the state. And yet, fundraising in this context has always been on a tightrope.

Sackey notes that whereas larger, mainstream organizations such as the Tate Gallery show a record of fundraising success, the same is not true for organizations dedicated to young Black artists: "Late at Tate Britain," for instance, is a curated program by the Tate Collective Producers, aged 15–25 years, who produce a range of free events and workshops for young people. Where they have had success attracting ongoing sponsorship, the same possibilities do not exist for Black and minority ethnic organizations:

Like the Tate, [the] "Late at Tate" [program], they get a grand association, it makes sense. . . . [But] in the last meeting I had with my Arts Council officer they said "You need to look at more sustainable models" and I said "What model? . . . What model have you seen where Black young people are getting funded by corporate or private donors, show it to me." (Interview with Nii Sackey, 2018)

Research in Canada (Murray & Hutton, 2012; Poyntz, 2018) about the challenges racialized and smaller youth arts organizations have competing for corporate sponsorship with larger, mainstream organizations buttresses Sackey's criticism. Black and minority ethnic organizations tend to operate as feeder sites for larger groups and industry, perhaps much in the way that Black arts and culture have long been appropriated and repurposed for larger mainstream culture success.

It is in this light that we argue that although contemporary forms of organization in a mixed economy show Black organizations competing relatively fairly, thus justifying the seeming fairness of the market, this is significantly untrue in respect of access to core public funding, which has, of course, provided years of public investment into non-Black organizations. Early on in its history, Bigga Fish received funding from ACE—for a set of turntables—and from Camden Council.

By the mid-2000s, its success led ACE to increase support through provision of nonprofit operational funding, helping it to become a leading YouthSite in the United Kingdom. At that time, it appeared to meet the objectives outlined by Bestwick above and demonstrated by the success of Roundhouse in respect of youth training in the cultural industries. By 2015, however, in the wake of the global financial crisis and a shift in government support for the arts under Conservative governments, Bigga Fish's operational funding was canceled and it was left in a precarious state. Bits of project funding continued from ACE, but the absence of a viable market alternative to support its work has produced a glass ceiling. Without sustained private support, Black and minority ethnic youth arts organizations are cast in an unenviable position: While working through and feeding commercial networks, those same networks produce barriers that limit and structure what Rupa Huq (2003, p. 197) has described as the "youth–cultural–commercial incorporation cycle." The limits of racial neoliberalism thus mark an important feature of a market-oriented system for managing social service agencies. Although invited to work with markets and in contract relationships with the state to mobilize and grow youth arts, these same structures impose limits on what key Black and minority ethnic organizations such as Bigga Fish can accomplish.

Resisting Institutionalization

It is important to view the emergence of other models of governance and financing in the youth arts sector in light of the experience of groups such as Bigga Fish. In Toronto, The Arts Mentoring Youth (AMY) Project launched in 2005 to support young female artists and actors living on the margins by taking them to plays and having conversations about artistic practice. Founders Claire Calnan and Pasha McKenley were encouraged to apply for project funding from Ontario Arts Council to develop theater programming for young women from underserved neighborhoods and those with a history in foster care in Toronto.

Ever since, AMY's program has focused on theater creation and mentorship. Other parts of the program have been added and include film, performance poetry, a program to support artists with disabilities, and a range of workshops for community groups, including transgender artists. AMY has provided food, transit tickets, and rehearsal space, and it has attempted to pay youth honoraria for their contributions.

Perhaps as kind of atavistic return to organizational forms from the 1960s and 1970s, AMY has always been a nonprofit with a minimal board of four directors and a larger team of coordinators made up almost entirely of BIPOC female and transgender youth. This structure emerged early in AMY's history and is focused on a youth-driven model of governance. Youth alumni and previous mentors in the program are recruited into leadership roles to provide continuity of experience for participants and a vision for the organization (see the life cycle histories in the Appendix for the not-uncommon challenge of sustainable legacy planning). AMY does not have operational funding, and in general, take-home pay for project directors has been modest. In 2014, both the Director and General Manager worked for 15 hours per week and earned CA$1,000 per month. Remuneration increased marginally in 2015, reflecting the organization's limited budget—less than CA$100,000 in 2015—and the fact that AMY has developed a reputation for frugal, flexible, and resourceful development.

This model of governance has enabled AMY to sustain its original political and social commitment, but it has also meant that it is constrained in its capacity and impact. AMY offers an example of the opportunity/limit "choice" organizations made or were forced to make: The stories of Ovalhouse, Roundhouse, Unity Charity, and Bigga Fish show the impact and challenges dominant modes of marketization and commercialization pose for groups, and The AMY Project reveals another side to this story. Although the organization has persisted and established a reputation for producing powerful work while supporting and mentoring young women, it always operates under the threat of financial ruin. It is challenged by small budgets, unsustainable levels of compensation, and dubious prospects for growth. As a form of assembly, its youth-centered model received praise from funders and other organizations in Toronto, and yet, without engaging the modes of market rationalization that have increasingly come to dominate the governance of YouthSites, AMY's future is tenuous. Again, the history of many organizations in the Appendix shows a distinct life course, rising and falling or being incorporated by other larger competitors. Amidst these cycles, however, the limits and boundaries of market rationalization and governance are significant.

In light of the challenges and complexities that have faced other organizational types, it is worth closing with Reel Youth in Vancouver, a platformed organization that is supported by a larger foundation, Tides Canada (now MakeWay!). Platform organizations are larger, often generic organizations that incubate projects until they can become financially self-supporting. This model of scaffolded growth is persistent in the third sector, right from origins in church-led youth clubs— SKETCH, for example, began as a platformed organization and now platforms others (see Chapter 8)—to more recent examples. Tides Canada provides overarching administrative support and oversight for social change projects such as Reel Youth, and although platformed organizations are perhaps not as common as a rational analysis might suggest, this model affords a mode of governance that encourages institutional agility, especially where public funding operates through a federated system, as in Canada.

Reel Youth started in Vancouver in 2005 as a community media empowerment project. Founding director Mark Vonesh left the finance industry and decided to work on a project using filmmaking and video production to support young people to speak up about social change. He began writing grants in 2004, and within the first year, Reel Youth was able to run 25 animation programs in Vancouver as well as a couple of production projects in remote communities. Soon afterwards, Reel Youth was approached by a series of communities and organizations to partner around media production programs for youth. That auspicious start has evolved to include collaboration with the Reel2Real International Film Festival, development of an innovative intergenerational program that brings together youth and seniors to produce videos about each other's experiences, and the creation of a series of social justice–oriented programs, including a small professional film production unit. In its opening decade, Reel Youth's work continued to be based in Vancouver, but by 2015, programs were offered in large and small communities throughout Canada and at international sites with local partners.

Tides Canada works with projects and community-based initiatives throughout Canada to provide structural support for operations and infrastructure. By being attached to Tides, Reel Youth can have offices in Toronto, Yellowknife, and Vancouver without requiring bricks-and-mortar spaces in each location. Rather, by being affiliated with Tides, it can sidestep the need to have permanent staff in Toronto and yet still apply for grants from local statutory authorities and foundations to carry out work throughout the province. For instance, it has carried out work in Brampton (in the greater Toronto area) and was able to get funding from the Ontario Trillium Foundation. The organization pays 10% of its annual revenues to Tides and in exchange receives support with payroll, back-end taxes, reporting on charitable status, human resources contracts, and service tax operations, as Vonesh explains:

> They do all the back-end charitable work that you know, needs to be done, but we're not really passionate about. I was asked to really focus on the program. Sure, we have to do administrative stuff for our programs, but I'm not worrying around about whether we're going to get our financials done in time for maintaining our charitable status. I don't have to you know, worry about you know, . . . creat[ing] our financial reports and it just allows me to focus on the actual work that I care more about. (Interview with Mark Vonesh, July 11, 2018)

Reel Youth has an advisory board, but it does not have any formal oversight. The compact model of Tides Canada has worked for Reel Youth and provides a point of major difference from other organizations in our study, many of which continue to spend time trying to secure funding for the back end of their operations.

While encouraging organizational agility, particularly in an environment that requires organizations to juggle multiple funding relationships and engage in sophisticated reporting practices, the model of platformed governance can be useful. It enables projects to remain lean, to focus on programming and future prospects rather than on administration and governance. This opens up potentially new funding lines and efficiencies. And yet, on the other hand, as evidenced by Reel Youth, the place-centered connections between platformed organizations and the communities they serve are thinner in comparison with those of many other organizations in the sector. The added value that organizations offer in terms of longevity and buildings, care, and relationships is more difficult without "mature" institutional form. Although Reel Youth began in Vancouver, its local "office" is, in fact, now located on Cortes Island (a small community outside of Vancouver). It has satellite locations in cities and towns throughout the country, but these locations do not exist in a traditional physical sense, even if Reel Youth operates in those communities. As a consequence, it is reasonable to conclude that Reel Youth's governance model provides the means for agility and efficiency, but it also splinters the deeper lines of connection that can emerge between the communities where young people live and the organizations that operate there.

Conclusion

This chapter has examined the complex forms of governance that have evolved in YouthSites. Questions about the governance of community-level organizations have typically been taken up in relation to an organization's governing body or board, with attention paid to board composition, the relationships between boards and management or staff, and board roles and effectiveness (Cornforth, 2012; Ostrower & Stone, 2006). In this chapter, we have investigated governance in the sector in relation to the structural conditions, types, and frameworks that define how YouthSites are organized and financed. We have shown how organizational structures and forms of assembly have operated, as well as the way finances and visual branding have served to enhance and challenge organizational stability, particularly when property has been proffered as the basis for sustainable futures. Together, the story of the "sector" is one of complex rationalization, where organizational structures have changed over time, where financing has required flexibility and sometimes a restructuring of organization mandates, and where growth is both compelling and deeply paradoxical.

We have been particularly vexed by the changing nature of the push and pull between funder and fundee in our sector. Contemporary forms of governance reward the enterprise of social actors, and, as we discussed in relation to Roundhouse or Unity Charity, organizations took up certain kinds of invitations in contradistinction to the older histories of state patronage and procurement that motivated, for example, the early days of Ovalhouse. The most explicit policy formulation of this push and pull of neoliberal governance in the third sector was the UK Conservative Party's "Big Society."[1] Coming into effect toward the end of our history, this pillar for the post-Thatcherite Conservatives of the 2010s trumpeted a form of social responsibility, civic participation, and communitarianism built on the kind of market-led, mixed economy third sector institutions exemplified by Unity or Roundhouse.

This vision was strictly regulated and driven by the key principles of new public management that began to take root in many countries from 1980s onwards. This chapter has explored how the history of the organizations exemplifies the perils, rewards, pains, and shape shifting as they learned to occupy what the discipline of new public management required from them. As part of the move to disaggregate organizations from the public sector to create quasi-autonomous groups (schools and hospitals, trusts for leisure, and recreation services, etc.) that are distinct from and yet responsible to government, the number of youth arts organizations has grown even if, like AMY, they sometimes struggle to sustain a future. New public management has also encouraged the development of quasi-markets in which the state acts as the "purchaser" of services from nonprofits that are to deliver services and compete with like organizations for this role (Cornforth, 2012). One powerful effect is a competitive environment in which youth arts groups—our examples are Roundhouse or Unity—are forced to compete with each other for new funding and associated contracts.

To monitor third sector activity, the state has come to rely increasingly on arm's-length means to monitor and manage nonprofit activities: " 'Performance-management' systems, including top-down target setting, service-level agreements, and strengthened regulatory, inspection and audit regimes" (Cornforth, 2012, p. 1120) have all become a regular part of operations and often in ways that force youth arts organizations to calibrate governance processes as part of managing key relationships with state, philanthropic, and other funding sources, as Bestwick argued in her telling of the history of Ovalhouse. As a result, the boundaries be-tween public, private, and third sector organizations have become increasingly blurred, leading to changes in older organizations and the rise of new hybrid groups. Organizations like Bigga Fish and Unity emerged in the early 2000s and are examples of a transition to social enterprises that compete in the marketplace and with states for contracts and services.

This is partly a move away from groups whose mandates address social, aes-thetic, and cultural change from within communities to groups that operate on a mixed economy model. YouthSites are in this way symptomatic of the unbundling of social services from the state and the rise of new third sector civic bodies that are now used to manage and support the provision of public services.

In general, most organizations in the youth arts sector are oriented around a *societal* purpose rather than financial goals, even if fiduciary responsibilities and issues of growth are ongoing concerns. A helpful way to distinguish YouthSites is by drawing on traditional distinctions between corporations, which are set up to create and distribute financial surpluses, and nonprofits, which are typically set up to serve broader social objectives (Wagner, 2015). Our organizations aimed to enhance the public good. New public management created a language to measure, manage, regulate, and deliver that good, and in many cases, we can see how histor-ically older forms of community value metamorphosed to take advantage of these opportunities. Organizations have clearly struggled to maintain their capacity to create societal value as a consequence of both internal dynamics and external, environmental conditions and relationships that groups must negotiate with youth, the state, markets, foundations, and others. In some cases, such as Bigga

Fish, the balance between enterprise and appropriation is perhaps uncomfortable, unsustainable, and unjust. Whether these forms of governance created the best opportunities for the communities they served, the best forms of arts practice, of learning, of educational opportunity, is a question we address in Chapter 10. Similarly, we need to ask in whose interests do the struggles to create institutions that we have documented here serve? There is much to admire in these stories of enterprise and market agility, but to what ends has all of this energy been put?

10

Conclusion

WHAT FUTURE FOR YOUTHSITES?

At the beginning of this book, we suggested that there was a shared arts-based informal, out-of-school practice with young people in the three cities we chose to study—London, Toronto, and Vancouver—that amounted to an administrative "sector" in the modern welfare state—a demarcated "field of practice" (Bourdieu, 1990). Chapters in Section 2 have offered characterizations of that practice—Chapter 5 on pedagogy and curriculum, Chapter 6 on community arts, Chapter 7 on forms of youth work, and Chapter 8 on modes of leadership. We have argued that these practices themselves derive from older traditions always present in the modern industrial and post-industrialized city. We have noted how forms of alternative pedagogy have their roots in progressivism developed at the turn of the 20th century (Amsler, 2015; Gerrard, 2016); how radical aesthetics derives from community arts (Crehan, 2011), popular theater, and critical pedagogy (Freire, 2000); and how traditions of care for marginalized young people even have their origins in sometimes radical forms of youth work (Griffin, 1993; Pollen, 2015; Shaffeeullah et al., 2020).

Early versions of youth arts were part of the post-war era, but the 1990s marked a period when this sector was "found" by the state and philanthropic organizations and constituted a viable resource to address a host of youth challenges, including the apparent failure of formal schooling to address the needs of socially disadvantaged youth and a requirement to prepare them for life as globally competitive subjects. What had been in some instances a movement of youth arts practices became a sector made up of organizations with distinctive and specific relationships with the state, philanthropic foundations, and civil society. We have located this sector within the changing dynamics of the city and have indicated the fractured, in-between urban spaces where key organizations have developed and sometimes thrived. These spaces are often the "leftover" zones in cities that have subsequently driven gentrification, and where new forms of securitization and changing models of creative economic

YouthSites. Stuart R. Poyntz, Julian Sefton-Green, and Heather Fitzsimmons Frey, Oxford University Press.
© Oxford University Press 2023. DOI: 10.1093/oso/9780197555491.003.0010

development have re-sorted where communities live and how resources are made available.

We have also suggested that it was the particularities of neoliberal governance—how welfare societies came to be reorganized—that enabled and constrained the growth, sustainability, and effectiveness of this sector. In general, we contend that these particularities led to the growth of a perpetually unstable sector in which organizational change, shifts in oversight and funding, changes in program priorities, and organizational geographies have been common features of a vital site of youth provision. A key part of this concluding chapter examines YouthSites in terms of the contradictions of neoliberalism while further reflecting on these tensions between opportunity and constraint, enterprise and audit, and radical care and welfare provision. Before that part of the discussion, however, we address three key challenges about the meaning of the "sector" as this emerged in our study. The chapter then looks beyond our contribution to the future of YouthSites in policy and practice.

Challenging Definitions

First is the challenge of *secificity* and *context*. For practical reasons, our study is rooted in three cities in England and Canada. In what ways do our cases represent a wider set of practices? Would the study have looked very different if we had used cases in the United States, Scandinavia, or Australia, for example? And in what ways are those practices peculiar to urban life in the Global North?

There are some studies of arts-based youth organizations not from the Global North—for example, Armenia (Sefton-Green, 2018), the Australian outback (Ladwig, 2018), Colombia (Brough, 2020), Bangalore (Ratnam & Vasudevan, 2018), and South Africa (Mitchell & Moletsane, 2018). Particularly because of challenges facing young people in the city, and in relationship to transitions between school and adulthood, many of the projects or activities captured in this range of literature do share common features. These include attitudes toward helping young people find a place in the city, express themselves, continue in their education, and, in circumstances in which they are excluded or marginalized (e.g., in relation to sexualities), be supported and recognized. There is a similar commonality in approaching the arts both as a resource for individual, community, and cultural expression and as a possible route toward employability and sometimes political engagement.

In the introduction to Section 2, we noted the body of literature analyzing work and organizations in the sector, mainly situated in the United States. Studies of "collegial pedagogy," voice, and civic activism (Soep & Chavez, 2010) sit alongside studies of neighborhood, community, and out-of-school support (Hirsch, 2005; McLaughlin, 1999, 2018; McLaughlin et al., 1994, 2009; Poyntz, 2018), with attention to the value of arts-based learning (Gallagher et al., 2020; L. Harvey et al.,

2002; Heath, 2012; Heath & Roach, 1999). There have been studies of youth development and activism (Kirshner, 2015; Poyntz, 2017) and sustained enquiry into the relationship of youth arts practice and opportunities in the creative and cultural industries (Campbell, 2013, 2019; Rennie, 2012; Rennie & Podkalicka, 2014; Watkins, 2019). In addition to all of these investigations, there are histories of youth clubs and other kinds of out-of-school/after-school education (B. Davies, 1999a, 1999b; Tyner, 2009), study of the work of relationality (DiGiacomo & Gutiérrez, 2015; Poyntz, 2021), and study of the role of the category of "youth" in the construction and management of the young in the city (Dillabough & Kennelly, 2010; Miles et al., 2002; Sukarieh & Tannock, 2015). We noted the attention given to the racial politics of provision in Bianca Baldridge's (2019) study of an after-school organization set in the northeastern United States. Similarly, work on youth arts and the politics of race and representation has informed our study (Butcher & Dickens, 2016; Crath, 2017; Leslie & Hunt, 2013; Monnet & Boukala, 2018).

All of the previously mentioned studies, from the Global North and beyond, are sensitive to contingencies and opportunities that arise out of local context. Across multiple sets of literature, the young people under discussion tend not to be part of a social or economic mainstream, and all are sensitive to the place-based horizons that seem to determine the possibilities for the young people in their city, often in contrast to national or global trends. Inevitably, local, community, regional, state, and national funding regimes are not equal, fair, or standardized in the ways that we might expect from studies of welfare provision or school systems.

However, the point of this summary at the end of our study is to underscore our argument that there is a persistent kind of institutional space across these types of youth provision. Not quite enough is known about this sector to make the case that it is a truly global phenomenon. However, like the neo-institutionalist studies of school and schooling (D. Baker, 2014; Meyer et al., 1997), which made the argument that the structure and form of the School have emerged as a touchstone institution in the modern bureaucratic state, we suggest that this sector, for all its partial visibility (see below), fulfills a similar structural and systemic form in the lives of many young people growing up in neoliberal cities around the world. These studies argued that the modern school shares an extraordinary range of common features in terms of structure of the day, the principles of curriculum, pedagogical traditions, physical location, professionalized workforce, credentialization, and so forth, and that these are now understood as the elements of a truly global system. By analogy, we suggest that for all the local differences and life opportunity contingencies for young people in the sector (which sometimes pretends not to be a sector), it nevertheless operates in a similarly structural fashion.

Sustaining this analogy is complicated by the fact that equilibrium is not a common feature of the sector. YouthSites have rather coalesced during a period of flux and transformation in relationships between the public sector, private life, and civil society (M. Warner, 2002). The role of civil society organizations, including nonprofits and other "social purpose organizations" (Greller, 2015,

p. 166), has expanded (D. Harvey, 2007; Lang, 2012), taking on roles in training, citizenship education, labor market development, social services, and so on that were once largely the remit of state or religious institutions or families. At the same time, the reach of markets and market-based institutions and practices has influenced how civil society organizations operate. In Chapters 7 and 9, we saw YouthSites working through economies of contract, fundraising, and branding, and Chapter 6 demonstrated how they often operate as incubators for cultural markets. Each of these developments highlights how organizations have moved away from what we might call a *movement-logic* to a *sector-logic* of administration and organization. Yet, as evidenced throughout this book, organizations simultaneously advocate for positive change; work to reduce barriers to participation, especially for socially excluded young people; and, in general, advocate for equitable and human-centered values. There is a third space quality to the sector (Soja, 1996; see also Oldenburg, 1989), of shifting boundaries, alliances, and tactics, where institutional moorings are tentative and where home and schooling have conjoined in a new space of social care. The geographer Edward Soja introduced an idea of a third space to describe a realm that is neither home nor school but, rather, a new kind of space. This is useful for thinking about YouthSites, which foster *youth scenes* and support *youth publics* but are also an administrative space of governance and care. Just as Julie Salverson (2011) characterized community-engaged theater, YouthSites "manages with maddening consistency to be vibrant with possibility, riddled with contradiction, and a messy quagmire of political and personal challenges—usually all at the same time" (p. vii).

Key to this argument, and our second main challenge, is the *relationship between practices and institutions*. This goes to the heart of whether we can make a case about the prevalence and depth of the sector. Although the chapters on education, arts, and youth (Chapters 5–7) examine activities and projects running across other fields and sectors, our approach to leadership and governance (Chapters 8 and 9), and, indeed, the whole thrust of our research described in Section 1 (Chapters 2–4) has been to emphasize the growth of projects into organizations and the aggregation of organizations into a sector. We do not suggest by this some simple process of institutional rationalization. As noted at various times throughout the book, the sector is, in fact, made up of a diversity of institutional forms—that is, nonprofits, extension programs, projects, and businesses—and in many ways this complexity is indicative of the way institutional rationalities common to the post-war welfare state era have given way to looser and more diverse forms in the age of neoliberal governance (Graham & Marvin, 2001). As a rule, YouthSites have not followed a straightforward logic of bureaucratization and stabilization leading to more extensive and sustainable relations with the state. Max Weber (1947) noted that both bureaucratization and professionalization are aspects of the modernization of society; in this sector, we contend these processes of institutionalization are engaged *conditionally*. Organizations answer to markets (and market-oriented state bodies) while proving their agility in response to a shifting set of social, technical, economic, and cultural challenges without expanding state institutions or the dependency of organizational clients on state allocation. In this sense, they embody a particular neoliberal institutional form.

Organizations in the sector have faced ongoing precarity. Their longevity seems to depend on their ability to leverage their role as locally effective, cost-efficient, and dynamic institutions. In turn, this relies on validation from both youth participants and the cultural workforce. Regularly responding to the shifting needs of a particular location and moment, and of individuals, organizations often make space for former youth participants to become staff. This makes innovation part of their business model, while simultaneously enacting a kind of sustainability through human resources–based institutional memory with an effect of perpetuating a community's valuing of the organization and itself. The fluidity and flexibility of organizations, nevertheless, become both an asset and a burden. To the extent that organizations are able to recalibrate their work, target populations, and attend to the inevitable conditions of risk, they are configured as innovators and leaders in comparison to traditional state-sponsored social service institutions, and yet, at the same time, they continue to encounter funding shortfalls and the need to reimagine their work in a manner that allows for little institutional stability.

Where complex forms of institutional rationalization characterize the sector, we have made the case that each organization or company (e.g., Ovalhouse Theatre in London and SKETCH in Toronto) has its own internal integrity while also being a constituent part within a larger system of governance shaped by new public management, welfare support, or educational remediation. We have been constantly intrigued by the tension between the way that the actors in organizations in our study have focused on the activities and practices they have carried out, even as it has been their struggle to form, consolidate, and continue to grow that has enabled such activities to become possible. We have recounted the history of the organizations in some ways as protagonists in their battles to achieve identity, security, and sustainability within an environment that seemed, as it were, so keen to give them oxygen at the same time as starving them of calories. For all the ways that systemic social needs in the three cities have been met with engagement and participation by young people and forms of monitoring and care, education, cultural and artistic development, and so forth, investing in the organizations in this sector has been precarious almost always to the point where the activities themselves are jeopardized.

This is why for all the weight of history, the shared traditions, the funding, the buildings, the life stories of so many people, even the systemic functions, we are aware that labeling this aggregate of activities a "sector" is still a tendentious claim. There may well be a political or ideological coherence behind the kinds of practices enacted by these institutions; they certainly all have strong points of correspondence along a continuum within which they can be found—for example, alternative schools, fringe theater, new media arts, and so forth. Nevertheless, without the kinds of diverse institutional spaces we have described, all of these practices would be impoverished. From a structural standpoint, the mainstream sectors require these hinterlands, these startups or incubators, in order to create the social cultural capital that enables other alternative kinds of growth to flourish (Campbell, 2013; Watkins, 2019). It is this systemic symbiotic relationship between the precarious organizations, their alternative practices, and more established cultural and economic forms that points to the category of sectoral or field identity at the heart of this book.

This brings us to our third challenge: the question of *status* and *visibility*. Chapter 2 especially focused on the methodological challenge we faced in locating, recording, and categorizing activities and organizations. We made the case that our study organizations could be seen as kinds of "analytic phenomena"—that is, they only emerged through the lens of our historical and contemporary enquiry. Yet, as Chapter 3 described (along with accounts in Chapters 6 and 8 in particular), many of the people and performances associated with YouthSites are high profile and attracted much publicity. As we wrote this final chapter, for example, the 2021 Oscar winner, British actor, Daniel Kaluuya acknowledged his early experiences at Weekend Arts College in London in many interviews. In Chapters 7 and 9, we noted how individuals or activities in this sector performed a rhetorical function within the micro-politics of race and representation, even if, at times, this created very difficult challenges for leaders and organizations.

In other words, the status and visibility of YouthSites seem to oscillate between extremes of high visibility (obviously Oscar winners are exceptional cases) and invisibility. This pattern is complicated by the way media panics about wayward youth, acts of youth violence, and youth alienation operate. In Chapter 1, we noted how the case of Reena Virk in 1997 in British Columbia generated concerns regarding youth gangs and violence among young women, leading indirectly to investment in organizations in the sector. The Yonge Street riot in Toronto in 1992 and the so-called Summer of the Gun in Toronto in 2005 eventually led to significant new funding for organizations such as Fresh Arts, Unity Charity, and The Remix Project to address youth alienation and tensions between the police and racialized youth. As public debate and media anxieties about young people have shifted during the 30 years of our enquiry, attention has turned to the sector as a kind of salve and means for constructively engaging with youth. Organizations have leveraged this attention for tactical ends to access funding and opportunity, especially in respect of the racial politics of representation. In the process, struggles over visibility have simultaneously taken on an ideological dimension.

In Chapter 2, we noted how a contestation over the representation of organizations and young people engages questions of power. We discussed how media panics highlight how media events bear on YouthSites' management of their own visibility. There is an aural pun in our terminology "YouthSite" with "youthsight," and this underpins this element of our contribution. Organizations in the sector depend on alignment with social policy and funding priorities, yet the relationship of the sector with these sources is vexed. Organizations need to be responsive to social policy, funding opportunities, and dominant media representations. Yet, in framing their visibility to others, organizations must be equally attuned to the differences between state, media, and philanthropic interests and the rights and needs of youth. This poses significant ideological challenges. Youth arts organizations have developed a language to describe who they are and who it is they work with. To negotiate this position, however, is to tread paradoxically between the demands of external funders and media representations and youth participants. As discussed in Chapters 2 and 4, labeling young people is a profound challenge for the sector because "deficit" labels that refer to patterns of "exclusion" and "vulnerability" risk pathologizing and "othering" the very youth the sector wishes to support. Yet this language serves to underscore the symbolic power of the sector among funders (Poyntz et al., 2019, p. 271), helping to uphold influential social structures and relationships. These dynamics can sit uncomfortably alongside notions of youth care within organizations. How organizations are made visible to others is thus as much about an ideological struggle over a language of representation that is fit for community and purpose, as it is about garnering attention and status.

Reviewing the history of organizations in the sector in respect of their struggles over visibility, we are inclined to think that the strange mixture of high-profile presence and invisibility, mediated through media panics, among other conditions, is a fit emblem for contemporary urban social provision. This structural context has shaped the sector as a third or in-between space. It has set the horizon within which everyday struggles over ideologies of youth representation have unfolded. The implication that this could therefore be a sector in which certain activities and organizations might benefit from more standardized investment—a professionalized workforce, audited curriculum, more equality of provision, and more monitoring—in order to avoid a feast-or-famine model of funding is one we take up in the final section of this chapter.

YouthSites and the Contradictions of Neoliberalism

In Chapter 1, we outlined four key contexts that have shaped this sector: the neoliberal state, education systems, the arts, and youth services. Not only do these fields or concepts provide contexts for the work of the organizations, but also, as we have suggested throughout, YouthSites themselves have driven a very particular kind of change and reform within each of these areas. Indeed, as Chapter 9 summarized, reviewing governance within a larger regime of control between public debate, the welfare state, entrepreneurial individuals, and a culture of social enterprise opened up extraordinary contradictions. We deliberately aimed to show change over a 30-year period (with our three census points sitting in the middle of decades of change), which, in both countries, encompassed periods of state control, welfare investment, and increased marketization in the provision of social or welfare services as well as changes in education and the arts.

The challenge of marking clear periods of time within this history has been important to us. We have particularly noted how 1995—our start date—looked backwards to forms of state-sponsored welfarism and community action even as the effects of globalization and the dismantling of welfare states changed the nature of the marketplaces for our study organizations. In Chapter 8, our account of leaders, we drew attention to the ways that individuals were formed by preceding generations of practice and how the impact of ideas unfolded out of time, as it were, as the leaders began to implement practices fostered in the 1970s within the opportunities created by competitive funding in the early 2000s. We also noted the development of new forms of leadership with a particular focus on a younger cohort who came of age in the mid-2000s and 2010s amid the realities of market-driven funding.

Our sense of periodization throughout the study has been very much influenced by the history of neoliberalism. By and large, neoliberalism is a catch-all label covering a number of social, political, and economic dimensions (Harvey, 2007). In drawing on this concept, we contend that YouthSites offer an exemplary focus to explore the meaning and impact of neoliberalism in social life. In a host of ways, youth have been a primary subject of neoliberalism. On one hand, the appeal in neoliberalism to notions of freedom, flexibility, global exchange, and consumerist lifestyles has long been cast in relation to global youth subjects (Kenway & Bullen, 2007). We noted in Chapter 7 on the city, for instance, how middle- and upper-middle-class youth identities have come to be linked with the development of creative cities, entrepreneurial energies, the consumer citizen, and so on. On the other hand, although neoliberalism offers the lure of a universal experience, nondominant, immigrant, and racialized youth have been a primary target of media anxiety, securitization, and social policy over three decades, standing as an emblem for the injustices of neoliberalism. We contend that YouthSites developed as a tactical force in response to these contradictions.

The very emergence of the sector was aided and necessitated by the pull-back of states from direct social services and welfare provision in the 1980s and 1990s, opening a space for new kinds of institutions and projects to emerge at the boundaries of civil society and public service. Over time, as we have noted, a market or private sector orientation came to dominate activity and funding. We have described this process as part of a larger dynamic of "unbundling" within cities that led to the disentangling of social services provision and infrastructure support from direct relations with the state and the development of a "messy" social field of youth provision (Graham & Marvin, 2001, p. 97).

Organizations in our sector leveraged this context for advantage by claiming space and articulating a public mission just as more traditional public institutions were in decline. In the main, youth arts organizations became social care structures, stand-in representatives, and scaffolding for young people that struggle against the institutionalization of their own advocacy. Through expressive forms—in voice, performance, media production, and visual art (see Chapter 6)—YouthSites have facilitated multiple participatory styles while combining on-the-ground connection and legitimacy with technical know-how. YouthSites are not counterpublics per se (M. Warner, 2002), whose primary focus is leading and mobilizing citizenry for political action. Sector organizations are rather better understood as civil society groups that advocate for, program to/with, and enable creative expression by those young people whose interests and needs are not addressed by traditional institutions.

A kind of feast-or-famine dynamic has haunted the sector, both fueling its growth and visibility and threatening its stability and future. The sector has expanded by casting light and creating opportunity for young people who have otherwise been ignored, demonized, or made subject to intense forms of regulation. But the arc of the sector in the three cities during the past three decades indicates that organizations have been squeezed as social provision under neoliberalism has been undercut by austerity, various forms of commodification (including, as we indicated in Chapter 9, the commodification of race), and the routing of social services through low-cost service delivery models.

In Chapter 9, we demonstrated how this has shaped the funding matrix of various organizations in the 2000s and 2010s. We also noted that the search for stability led some groups (i.e., Ovalhouse, Paddington Arts, and Roundhouse Studios) to develop their own property in the hope that this would help steady the organization for the foreseeable future. In the context of neoliberalism, however, such tactical moves are vexed. Our own and related research (Lang, 2012; Poyntz, 2017; Poyntz et al., 2019) demonstrate that when organizations have to pursue a diversity of funding sources, they tend to cede control to funders because the pressure to produce increasingly more applications encourages organizations to initiate programs to serve the grant rather than the organizations' fundamental aims. The specificity and force of an organization's advocacy then risk becoming diluted (Lang, 2012, pp. 70–72). And, although property ownership has been advantageous, organizations with buildings have often had to rent out their space and limit their own activities in order to survive.

Amid these tensions, YouthSites have nonetheless demonstrated how care structures (Scannell, 2014) can be sustained in the context of neoliberalism. We borrow this notion of care structure from Paddy Scannell (2014), who defines these structures as the resources, systems, and concepts that scaffold our lives in ways that allow us to accomplish the ends we hope for. YouthSites create conditions of care for youth participants, sometimes for young people's families, and often for their facilitators and mentors. In Chapter 4, on youth experience, and in Chapter 8, on leaders, we noted the multiple ways radical and ongoing forms of care operate across the sector. While offering technical training, skills development, and sometimes brand promotion, YouthSites have provided a fulsome range of care. As discussed in Chapters 2, 3, 7, and 8, organizations commonly provide access to safe spaces, stability and nutrition, support for minor travel costs, various life skills (e.g., self-confidence and validation), opportunities for community culture change, creative materials, and flexible open-access programming. Distinctive pedagogies provide rigorous technical skills and training, in addition to mentoring, access to social capital (including professional and celebrity networks), and transitions to further training. Credentials are not uncommon in the sector, but they are not the focus. Rather, care for the whole human is the priority. Leaders are radically committed to young people, as described in Chapter 8. Feminized care structures in the sector typically work to counter the instrumentalization of people and the exclusion of opportunity for nondominant youth, which can often be the experience of more mainstream institutions. Leaders such as Phyllis Novak of SKETCH are conscious of their own privilege and have worked to support programs that disrupt the reproduction of power and exclusion. Meg Solis of Miscellaneous Productions suggests there was no "catch" in the way support has been provided. Rather, care structures in the sector reflect a culture of concern and attention, patience, and, often, radical hope. Certainly, these structures and practices have been compromised by twists and turns in funding, by the rise of oversight and audit cultures, by shifting fears of the young, and by other tendencies common to neoliberalism. Yet, as we contended in Chapter 7, the sector has kept on with it, making a social and culture space in civil society that offers stability for young people to orient out into a world that can often seem stark.

What Futures for YouthSites?

If any one single emotion accompanied our enquiry during the past 4 years, it is the sense of hope noted above. Like an anthem or a phrase, it is impossible to get out of our heads the optimism, positivity, and forward-looking-ness in the organizations we encountered. Given a key part of so many of these organizations' missions derived from creating opportunities for the young people who had been failed by so many other people and systems in their lives, the sense of possibility, the belief in opportunity, and a sheer hope for change seemed to animate people and places across all three cities.

This, in turn, creates an ethical dilemma for us. As we disentangled the grim functioning of markets and the, at times, cynical attitudes toward policy for youth, how do we square our intellectual pessimism with this heartfelt optimism? Furthermore, in this final section, we want to look forward. We want to ask what the history recounted in this book might suggest for the future of these organizations and for the kinds of practices we have excavated. What hope for this hope? In responding to these questions, this final section offers a series of short points looking forward and challenging policymaking for young people mainly aimed at countries in the Anglo-American orbit.

THE DIGITAL VERSUS PLACE AND PRESENCE

At an event organized to commemorate the 10-year anniversary of the London-based Supporting Talent to Enterprise Programme (STEP) initiative, described in Chapter 1, a number of younger organizations made the point that forms of digital sociality and, indeed, the whole growth of friendship and participation online has changed the purpose and role of organizations whose primary rationale was that they could bring people together. The balance between togetherness and isolation, community and solitude, is, of course, complex, but there is no doubt that much current research into the social and community life of young people is focused on all kinds of online experiences and interactions (Ito et al., 2010).

Many YouthSites are highly digital, from using social media and web presence to creative work with digital technology in music and media production. However, the extent to which a YouthSite is now faced with a move online is a key question for youth policy. Although there are many forms of online participation, especially through gaming (Ito et al., 2018), does this signal the end of bringing people together in face-to-face situations? What would be lost and gained from such a move? And how do new forms of YouthSites negotiate with this kind of competition?

As we consider these questions, we argue that dissolution of in-person, shared spaces is undesirable. Online spaces extend options for youth engagement (Keller & Ringrose, 2014) rather than replace them. Although the COVID-19 pandemic demonstrated ways online engagement opens up opportunities for young people who would not be able to participate in conventional on-site experiences (for mental health, distance and transportation, physical disability, or other reasons), some young people clearly assert that "collaborating through a screen does not hold the same experience as an in-person collaboration would" (Haley, quoted in Fitzsimmons Frey & Kerekes, 2021). Shared spaces, meals, relationships, care, communities, and the ambiances mentioned earlier are all facets of the co-presence possible in YouthSites. Online experiences invite young people in. They create inclusive experiences for those who could not otherwise participate, and they extend engagement for those who would like to participate, both online and on-site. They will not disappear, and going forward youth arts organizations are likely to find themselves programming for both online and on-site experiences.

At the same time, the history of the organizations recounted in this book revolves around the challenges of a physical resource being made available to specific populations who are addressed and welcomed into certain places. We have told the history of place-based arts performance, of care and home. Some commentators will interpret the current role of online existence only as even greater evidence for the need for organizations that we have described; others look to cut costs and create new kinds of blended institutions. Chapters 4 and 8 in particular have attempted to show how time, relationships, and people impact on youth to 'work their magic in these kinds of contexts'. They also make the case that substantial economic and social investment produces particular kinds of socially beneficial effects, but that the consensus about the need to provide such investment is fast dissipating. As the generation of people formed in the 1970s and 1980s exits the labor market, how younger generations schooled in different cultures of connection and communication take center stage is an exciting challenge. Digital platforms have no doubt extended the reach, viability, and program offerings of organizations in the sector, but we contend that the digital on its own cannot sustain the experience of togetherness and connection made possible by the affective cultures of place in YouthSites. The smell, feel, and semiotics of YouthSites enable young people to gather, to be seen and heard, and to find others. At their best, YouthSites are durable places of trust and belonging in fragmented and inequitable societies. We worry that the appeal to austerity and flexible online program delivery frameworks risks erasing these features of YouthSites, leaving behind a more precarious and vulnerable sector.[1]

PROFESSIONALIZATION AND STANDARDIZATION

One solution to the problem of capricious funding would be for the sector to become its own domain instead of performing the function of "filling in" between other sectors. This goes to the paradox of the non-formal sector (Sefton-Green, 2013). It is precisely because of its capacity to act outside of full schooling, conventional arts, and so forth that these organizations can reach their constituencies; but without degrees of permanence and longevity, they cannot always continue to be as effective. One possible future for work undertaken by the sector would be for the organizations to move away from a client-led and project-driven structure to become more established within "departments" of youth services, the arts, and education. This would, in turn, necessitate a different approach toward the training and credentialization of the workforce and the standardization of recruitment and delivery practices. The institutionalization of the sector would then become complete, but at what cost?

There are parts of the world where some of these activities are institutionalized in this fashion. We especially identify the northern European and Scandinavian youth work tradition here. The idea of youth-oriented pedagogy, management, and teaching has been far more embedded in the range of state and privately funded institutions, from youth clubs in large cities to "folk" schools in Scandinavia. Scholarship informs and validates practice (Erstad et al., 2016; Gilje, 2012; Gilje & Groeng, 2015; see also Chapter 7, this volume), forms of youth culture (Fornas et al., 1995), and, indeed, theories of learning particular to the youth context (Nissen, 2012). Qualifications and credentials and academic study are part of the bargain between secure funding and institutionalization.

With this context in mind, it is not difficult to anticipate a creeping professionalization of the sector we have analyzed in North America and the United Kingdom. Baldridge's (2019) study makes the point that pressures to support school-defined formal learning outcomes determined practices in the organization she studied, which in turn had consequences for the racialization of governance and some of the tensions between the ways that the values of Black workers and leaders became conflicted. In Chapter 8, we focused on key leaders and mentors but did not account for the very high numbers of underemployed artists and youth workers who consistently pick up part-time employment in organizations in the sector and who are often valued for their expertise and experience rather than simply their credentials. In other words, the kinds of traditions and approaches during the past 30 years that we reviewed might well be subject to change if cities in the Global North decide to invest in this sector structurally. Without care, investment in the sector could reinforce barriers to participation in arts and youth work and accelerate financial precarity, so that standardizing the work in ways that could have unintended side effects. As explained in Chapters 7 and 8, when youth participants become facilitators, trained through experience, apprenticeship, or mentorship-type models, they help establish a powerful community of care that highlights positive possibilities for youth. If cities choose to invest in YouthSites, we suggest they certainly need different kinds of "changemaker" leadership that, as Mike Murawski (2021) explains, is human-centered, collaborative, and practically focused on equity and relationships.

Throughout this book, we have paid attention to the functions that YouthSites might have within existing institutional arrangements. In Chapter 5, we discussed ways that they might work as safety valves and/or research and development incubators for correcting system failings and for reform; in Chapter 6, we examined how arts practices and disciplines might embody different kinds of alternative social arrangements. The challenge of professionalization can also be seen in terms of what role we anticipate the sector will play with regard to these broader social functions. As collective authors, we note that this is one of the few points in the book where we might disagree with each other. Some of us focus on the possibilities for sectoral reform, whereas others are horrified at this prospect; some think it is the only rational way for the sector to continue, whereas others believe it would signal its death. This is not just a question of individual optimism or pessimism. It also highlights the difficulty of discerning longer term institutional trajectories—of knowing how trends predict futures. It was a 1985 study of community organizations, *What a Way to Run a Railroad: An Analysis of Radical Failure* (Landry et al., 1985)—a study of dashed ideals and dysfunctional leadership in community arts—that inspired the application for funding that led to this book.

We hoped that by excavating the history of these organizations during the past 30 years, we might avoid repeating systematic challenges for workers and practitioners—what some scholars have labeled policy or institutional amnesia (Alastair & Brian, 2019)—so that understanding broader social functions carried out by these organizations might help focus on quality practice and governance. Of course, predicting trends is not the same thing as creating other possible futures, so we remain open to the challenge of whether professionalization and standardization are both desirable and/or necessary or inevitable. This is a challenge for future work.

IMPACTS AND EFFECTS

One consequence of an absence of professionalization of this sector is that there is a shortage of university departments providing accreditation and, therefore, a relatively small amount of scholarship in the area. This does not diminish the texts referred to in this book, nor does it discount universities that have developed specialist research centers in out-of-school learning; indeed, we have already mentioned the academic traditions in social pedagogy in northern Europe. However, most writing and study of this sector take the form of commissioned research reports that can be found in the "gray literature." In Chapter 2, we mentioned the difficulty of interpreting many accounts of practice in the sector because of the partial or instrumental nature of the evaluations or assessments. This question of how the sector represents itself to wider stakeholders through publicity or, indeed, to key funders in the form of annual reports also emerged as a point of tension in Chapter 9 when we discussed governance.

The dominant mode of the gray literature is *evaluative*. Reports seek to measure and value activity using a wide range of metrics, theories of impact, descriptors of effect, and diverse methods of accounting. There are no shared warrants—indeed, how could there be given the lack of institutional conformity or bureaucratic rationale? If activities in this sector continue to consolidate, if organizations continue to institutionalize, then a greater understanding about what counts and how to count it will develop as a shared norm. Here, we have argued that a necessary diversity of practice bringing together arts and education, care and place, participation and welfare has made it difficult for norms to grow and for common metrics to be accepted as meaningful universal measures.

This is not to say that much of the gray literature—and we note that much of it is produced by academics working in a consultative capacity—does not aspire to establish relevant and purposeful indicators that can have traction with all stakeholders. We could point, for example, to the work of the Big hART initiative/organization,[2] which has produced a series of evaluations theorizing and then offering practical ways to assess impacts relating to health and well-being, community development and creative spaces, the development of agency and a sense of efficacy, the use of participatory arts for an expressive life, strengthening capacities and dispositions for learning, and the reinvention of identity through cultural practices. There is no question that this kind of agenda would have been part of day-to-day discussions within organizations and between them and their funders over the period of time and across the countries we have described in this book. Similarly, innovative, theoretically informed models to document and assess learning that is sensitive to the informal and media-rich environments of YouthSites (Lemke et al., 2015) are indicative of an intellectual culture of reflection that is part and parcel of the history we have told in this book. Our challenge, however, is not to design new kinds of evaluation but, rather, to ask these organizations how and in what ways adhering to norms and conventions in what counts as good or high-quality non-formal learning or community arts practice might count for them, their funders, and the communities they serve.

On a final note, the organizations we have explored exist because of the young people who crave opportunities, resources, and training to make inspiring creative work that is meaningful to them. In a very real way, the *sector* exists because of social, government, and institutional networks that enable the dedicated people who are listening to young people to address demands. Because the demand is youth driven (even as adults offer provision and care), the ways the organizations address the arts and young people continue to shift with their interests, needs, and concerns. This question and the ones we asked about the role of place-making in the digital age, as well as our speculation about the knock-on effects from increasing standardization, are ones that a mature sector would ask. YouthSites now sit at a crossroads in societies beginning to organize forms of everyday life and economic production in frighteningly hostile environments. Young people will bear the highest costs for changes in climate and social order. This book is testimony to the thousands of people who have tried to offer young people, often lost in our modern cities, hope, practical guidance, and meaningful experience. That challenge will continue, whatever form it takes.

APPENDIX

List of Organizations

Organization	City	Date Founded (and Date of Termination, if Relevant)	Turnover 2015 (and over Period)	Number of Students 2015 (and over Period)	Governance Structure	Key Funders 2015
7th Generation Image Makers	Toronto	1996	"From an $80,000 budget with two staff to an Agency of 180 staff and a service budget of over $20 million"*	"Graduated 15 youth from various accreditation programmes"; "served 10,633 meals"	Part of Native Child and Family Services—charity	Ministry of Children and Youth Services
Access to Media Education Society (AMES)	Vancouver	1996	$128,667 (2004: $291,681)	"The process of consulting with over 450 young immigrants is in full swing" (2004 annual report, p. 4); "40 teachers/ classrooms, 700 elementary students, 300 elders and community members, and 40 artists in the Lower Mainland and on the southern Gulf Islands" (2015 annual report, p. 4)	Charity	Arts Council, VSB, Vancouver Foundation, City of Van, Vancity, Telus (2015 annual report, p. 1)
Access to Music Foundation	Vancouver	2005	$79,273 (2011: $32,582)	"Since [2010], we have become a leader in supporting music education by putting instruments into the hands of thousands of music students across the province, encouraging hundreds of young people to express themselves through songwriting, and assisted many gifted young artists in the next stage of their careers" (website)	Charity	"Is supported through generous individual and corporate donations and private foundations. Our public fundraising efforts include an annual gala, concerts, third party events and social media campaigns. Access to Music Foundation is a charitable organization" (website)

Type of Student 2015	Property/ Residences 2015 (and over the Period)	Neighborhood (and Character Change over the Period)	Mission 2015	Art Forms 2015	Programs/Mode of Delivery 2015	Accreditation/ Links with Formal Education Providers 2015 (and over the Period)
"Native people," "at risk youth", "artists"	Native Youth Resource Centre	Downtown	"We provide ongoing accessible and quality fine art instruction taught by professional contemporary Native artists, mentors and Elders"; "Committed to providing quality and accessible art programming in a culturally supportive and safe environment"	Visual arts, Indigenous arts, film	Ongoing instruction, public art commissions, community partnerships	Some programs with high school accreditation
"AMES programs primarily engage young people with lived experiences of various forms of oppression. Connecting with youth also means engaging the adult allies—artists, educators, activists, mentors and community workers—who support them" (AMES website)	Lower Mainland and Southern Gulf Islands	"Amplif[ies] and extend[s] the reach of youth visions and views, increase[s] awareness about issues that matter, spark[s] dialogue and foster[s] imaginative visions for change"	Film and media	Guided by community-based artists and mentors; in-school and after-school programs	None
With a talent or passion for music, vulnerable youth	Lower Mainland		"to enhance leaning opportunities for young artists and to help vulnerable youth find their place in society"	Music	School partnerships	None

(continued)

Organization	City	Date Founded (and Date of Termination, if Relevant)	Turnover 2015 (and over Period)	Number of Students 2015 (and over Period)	Governance Structure	Key Funders 2015
Apples and Snakes	London	1982	£714,369 (1995: £103,832; 2005: £574,468)	"[N]early 30,000 people who have benefited from our renowned participation and outreach programmes"(2015 annual report)	Charity	ACE; multiple LAs; European Social Fund, Trusts and Foundations—BBC Children in Need, Tuxien Foundation, John Lyon's Charity, City Bridge Fund, the Monument Trust, Esme Fairbairn, Paul Hamlyn, John Ellerman Foundation (2005: ACE, Trusts and Foundations—Esme Fairbairn, Association of London Government, Creative Partnerships) (1995: multiple LAs, Deptford City Challenge, London Arts Board; London Borough Grants Scheme)
ArtHeart	Toronto	1991	$222,145		"Not-for-profit charitable organization"	Other charities
Arts Umbrella	Vancouver	1979	$5,464,245 (2011: 4,984,616) (annual reports)	20,063 students (2014–2015); 2011: 24,000 (annual reports)	Charity	Fundraising, government, corporate, foundations

Type of Student 2015	Property/ Residences 2015 (and over the Period)	Neighborhood (and Character Change over the Period)	Mission 2015	Art Forms 2015	Programs/Mode of Delivery 2015	Accreditation/ Links with Formal Education Providers 2015 (and over the Period)
"Children and young people in school and college"; "vulnerable young people outside mainstream education"; "emerging artists"	Office space within The Albany Performing Arts Centre; that venue also used for performances	London/ national	"Produc[es] exciting, engaging and transformative work . . . giving a voice to those whose creativity is suppressed"	Spoken word	Projects with schools, libraries, prisons and hospitals; artist mentoring; commissioning and touring	None
"Children, youth and adults in inner-city Toronto"	"Part of a dynamic arts and cultural centre"; 'Daniels Spectrum Artscape': 1,800 square foot art studio; computers, washroom, books, arts supplies; rented (moved from 40 Oak Street in 2004 ("humble beginnings in this church basement")	Regent Park, within Canada's original and largest Government Housing Project; "ArtHeart continues to be an anchor in a community going through dramatic change and revitalization"	"Supportive environment for children, youth, and adults in inner-city Toronto with access to free art studio space, instruction and supplies"; "To empower our participants to improve their quality of life"	Visual arts	Studio arts; food for participants; youth employment; "The program increases the ability of youth to earn and maintain a living while teaching appropriate attitudes and behavior needed in the workplace" (twelve 14- to 17-year-olds trained per year)	None
Ages 2–19 years		Surrey and Vancouver	"Builds community and delivers profound life experiences . . . inspire[s] people to live creative, authentic, and courageous lives"	Visual art, performing arts, media	Ongoing instruction; workshops; class based	None

(continued)

Organization	City	Date Founded (and Date of Termination, if Relevant)	Turnover 2015 (and over Period)	Number of Students 2015 (and over Period)	Governance Structure	Key Funders 2015
Art Starts	Toronto	1993	$788,843		Charity	
ArtStarts in Schools Society	Vancouver	1996	$3,029,359 (2012: $1,297,994; 2005: $149, 119)	2015: 18,868 participated in projects (2005: involving more than 10,000 young people, booked 250 events in schools) (annual reports)	Charity	British Columbia Arts Council, Vancouver Foundation, City of Vancouver
Artec	London	1980s–1990s	1997: "just under £1,000,000" (Source: *The Independent*)	"Intensive training"	Part of Islington LA	Islington LA, Arts Council, European Union

Type of Student 2015	Property/ Residences 2015 (and over the Period)	Neighborhood (and Character Change over the Period)	Mission 2015	Art Forms 2015	Programs/Mode of Delivery 2015	Accreditation/ Links with Formal Education Providers 2015 (and over the Period)
"Vulnerable people"; "underserved and stressed communities"			"Inspires and cultivates social change by bringing professional artists and Toronto residents together to create community-building art projects in all artistic disciplines for underserved and stressed communities"; "providing a safe, supportive and inclusive environment for self-expression and creative collaboration"; "using the arts to help end the negative cycles associated with marginalization and poverty"	Multi arts		None
Kindergarten to Grade 12	Gallery, dark rooms, office space that is rented out—building granted by ACE in 2003 and opened in 2007 (previously a small cinema and production workshop at nearby location)	Throughout British Columbia	"Transform[s] the way children and youth are engaged, in and through the arts, and . . . promot[es] the value of the arts in young lives"	Multidisciplinary arts	Artist in classrooms; performances	None
"Local young people who are new to technology but have creative talent" (*The Independent*)	Based in local government building	Islington (Index Multiple Deprivation rank of average rank 2015: 13; 2000: 8) (68% White— 2011 census)	"Offer[s] training for employment in the burgeoning digital media industries to people who might not usually access these opportunities"	Digital media	"Although set up originally to offer training to socially excluded groups in digital media, it diversified practice and worked as an artists' lab, a production house, a training centre for professionals and an innovation centre" (Sefton-Green, 2008, p. 5)	None

(continued)

Organization	City	Date Founded (and Date of Termination, if Relevant)	Turnover 2015 (and over Period)	Number of Students 2015 (and over Period)	Governance Structure	Key Funders 2015
Bigga Fish	London	2001			Not-for-profit social enterprise	ACE, Mayor of London, trusts and foundations
Children's Peace Theatre	Toronto	1996	$330,000 (2005: $250,000)		Charity	Trilium, Arts Council
CircusWest	Vancouver	1984	$923,415 (2012: 657,081)	Since 2003, it has grown six times in size (old website)	Charity	Fee for service; government funding (no annual reports available—based on Canada Revenue Agency)

(continued)

Type of Student 2015	Property/Residences 2015 (and over the Period)	Neighborhood (and Character Change over the Period)	Mission 2015	Art Forms 2015	Programs/Mode of Delivery 2015	Accreditation/Links with Formal Education Providers 2015 (and over the Period)
"Disadvantaged young people"; "inner-city youth"; "young Black and ethnic minorities"	Office space in The Trampery (many previous bases—both alone and hosted in arts centers, etc,, including one large building that itself hosted other organizations)	London/national	"Work[s] to address the significant problem of the lack of resources and opportunities for inner city youth . . . provide[s] high quality performance and work opportunities to young creatives"	Music	Ongoing "street teams" and leadership programs; discrete projects such as tours; tailored projects for other youth organizations	None
Indigeneity; "people with a passion for social change"	Since 2007, below market rate rent	East Toronto	"Uses the arts and artistic creativity as critical tool for personal and social transformation"; "a catalyst for ideas, discussions and actions that make the arts more central and meaningful to people's lives, in order to promote healthier young people, more vibrant democracies and equitable societies"; "where young people can create and learn from Elders"	Theatre, drama	Year-round programming for young, Indigenous style "subversive" youth leadership with elder support; Speak your Peace Festival; microgrants; Dear Native Youth; Black Youth; Conflict Transformation workshops in schools	None
Have offered ACRIX classes to teach introductory skills to at-risk youth in Vancouver (website); ages 3–19 years	East Vancouver		"Develop[s] skills in circus arts and performance, while increasing . . . fitness and self-confidence in a safe and fun environment"	Performing arts	Workshops; classes; performance-based work	None

(continued)

Organization	City	Date Founded (and Date of Termination, if Relevant)	Turnover 2015 (and over Period)	Number of Students 2015 (and over Period)	Governance Structure	Key Funders 2015
Community Music (CM)	London	1983	£542,959 (2005: 536,455; 1995: £323,426)		Charity	Youth Music; Haringey LA; ACE (2005: London Arts Board; Association of London Government; European Social Fund; Southwark LA; London Metropolitan University; Youth Music; London Development Agency) (1995: London Arts Board; London Borough's Grant Scheme; multiple LAs; European Social Fund; trusts and foundations)
Collage Arts	London	1985	£2,026,986 (1995: £172,083; 2005: £1,426,744)		Youth program running as part of larger "arts development, training and creative regeneration charity"—charity	Big Lottery Fund; Skills Funding Agency (1995: European Social Fund; Haringey LA; Foundation for Sport and Arts)

Type of Student 2015	Property/ Residences 2015 (and over the Period)	Neighborhood (and Character Change over the Period)	Mission 2015	Art Forms 2015	Programs/Mode of Delivery 2015	Accreditation/ Links with Formal Education Providers 2015 (and over the Period)
"Local young people"; "at risk"; "from beginner to professional"	Purpose-built studios and theater linked to Brady Arts and Community Centre (originally an attempt to build a National Jazz Centre in a warehouse in Covent garden funded by the Greater London Council, which never opened). Space in Clerkenwell, 1992–	Tower Hamlets (Index Multiple Deprivation rank of average rank 2015: 6; 2000: 1) (45% White— 2011 census)	"Offer[s] a diverse and exciting programme of courses, live events and professional training. This includes a foundation degree in music production and business, instrumental and music production tuition"	Music	Ongoing workshops and rehearsal space; ongoing instrument tuition; showcasing and live events; professional development for musicians and community leaders	Foundation Degree in Music Production and Business; City and Guild accredited course "Music Leader" (1995: NVQs; course accredited by London Metropolitan University)
"Creative individuals with inquisitive and entrepreneurial minds"; "NEET"	Recording studio, digital training spaces, plus studio buildings hosting "a community of over 250 artists and creative businesses" acquired over the life of the organization (1995: digital recording studio, artists studios) (2005: Chocolate Factory Studios 1 & 2 and training unit)	Haringey (Index Multiple Deprivation rank of average score 2015: 21; 1999: 10) (61% White—2011 census)	"A vibrant centre in the creative industries where people from all social backgrounds can participate"	Media, design, music	Short weekend courses; accredited courses; employability program for NEET 18–24; exhibitions and festivals	Creative Apprenticeship Diploma in Creative and Digital Media; BTEC in Creative and Digital Media (1995: Music Business course accredited by Middlesex University; City and Guild Sound Engineering course accredited by College of North East London)

(continued)

Organization	City	Date Founded (and Date of Termination, if Relevant)	Turnover 2015 (and over Period)	Number of Students 2015 (and over Period)	Governance Structure	Key Funders 2015
Create Jobs	London	2009		"In 2015–16 Create Jobs engaged 500 young people and helped 100 into employment, through its programme"	A program run by two other arts organizations: A New Direction (AND) and Create—both charities. AND has close links to ACE	Mayor's Fund for London; Job Centre Plus; trusts and foundations—Garfield Western Foundation, Bloomberg Philanthropies
CUE	Toronto	2008	$250,000–$300,000 (2008: $44,000)	"Directly supported 78 artists in project creation"; "40 young people engaged in a variety of leadership positions"	Began as project of SKETCH and operates on a shared platform with it	Trillium; Toronto Arts Council; Toronto Arts Foundation; SKETCH; Platform
Four Corners	London	1973	£370,696 (1995: £108,683; 2005: £428,017)	500 users of training program	Charity	ACE; European Union; Creative Skillset; trusts and foundations (2005: Arts Council England; European Social Fund; National Lottery; Foundation for Sports and Arts)

Type of Student 2015	Property/Residences 2015 (and over the Period)	Neighborhood (and Character Change over the Period)	Mission 2015	Art Forms 2015	Programs/Mode of Delivery 2015	Accreditation/Links with Formal Education Providers 2015 (and over the Period)
"Less advantage socio-economic groups"; "local young people aged 16–24 who are not in education or training"	None—run by the organization A New Direction in its office space in Old Street; programs take place in different settings across London	London	"Aims to bring more 16–24 year-olds from . . . [particular] boroughs into the creative sector, diversifying the workforce and providing beneficial experiences for both employers and job-seekers"	Design, digital design	Intensive courses; mentoring; work placements and employment brokering	None ("We co-design industry based training with top employers")
"New generation artists who live and work on the margins"; "artists who experience marginalization, face systemic barriers, and who have been excluded by conventional arts and cultural institutions"; "artists of colour"; "artists [who] identified mental health issues as a barrier to their artistic careers"	None	Citywide	"A high-access funding program offering not only financial support for art projects, but also consultation in preparing project proposals, support throughout the production process, and opportunities for public exhibition"	Visual arts, writing, craft, multi arts	Funding and mentorship; outreach partnerships with arts and community organizations	None
"Disadvantaged young adults"; "unemployed"; "groups currently under-represented in the industry—those who are BAME, female, disabled and/or from disadvantaged backgrounds"	Gallery, dark rooms, office space that is rented out—building granted by ACE in 2003 and opened 2007 (previously a small cinema and production workshop at nearby location)	Tower Hamlets (Index Multiple Deprivation rank of average rank 2015: 6; 2000: 1) (45% White—2011 census)/London	"Empower[s] and enable[s] the creative talents of people . . . by providing access to high-quality affordable facilities and equipment"	Film and photography	Filmmaking training, mentorship, and employment advice	College Network/Skillset accredited courses (2005: London Open College Network accreditation)

(continued)

Organization	City	Date Founded (and Date of Termination, if Relevant)	Turnover 2015 (and over Period)	Number of Students 2015 (and over Period)	Governance Structure	Key Funders 2015
Frames Film Program	Vancouver	2012			An off-site program of Frog Hollow Neighbourhood House	
Green Thumb Theatre	Vancouver	1976	$861,820 (2010: $1,123,313)	"Performing for more than 50,000 children" (website)	Charity	Government; corporate; foundations
Instruments of Change	Vancouver	2012	$66,000		Charity	Benefit events; private donations; Tides; City of Vancouver; Indiegogo campaign; Canada Council
Intersections Media	Vancouver	2014	$502,006		Charity	Government; corporate; foundations
Kapisanan	Toronto	1980s	$137,000	Five or six on each program	Charity— partnership with SKETCH	Toronto Arts Council; Ontario Arts Council; ArtReach Toronto

Type of Student 2015	Property/ Residences 2015 (and over the Period)	Neighborhood (and Character Change over the Period)	Mission 2015	Art Forms 2015	Programs/Mode of Delivery 2015	Accreditation/ Links with Formal Education Providers 2015 (and over the Period)
Multi-barriered youth (ages 16– 30 years)	Operating out of East Vancouver's Drive Youth Employment Services (D-YES)	East Vancouver	"Provides opportunities for youth to learn the basics of filmmaking in a supportive, safe and fun environment"	Media	Each 10-week cycle involves weekly lessons and two shooting and editing weekends	None
Young audiences	Owns a studio space, available for rental	National	"A way for young people to reflect on the kinds of issues that they may be curious about or grappling with themselves, but don't feel comfortable broaching in a traditional classroom setting"	Theater	Performance; touring	None
"Diverse"		East Vancouver	"Uses the arts as an educational tool to empower people to become instruments of transformative change in their own lives"	Music	Community collaboration	None
Face barriers to employment and/or education; ages 19–30 years		East Vancouver	"Offers an employability and life skills workshop and work experience opportunity to youth facing multiple barriers to employment, and . . . seeking employment in the film and television production industry"	Media	Workshops	None—but there is compensation
"Filipino-Canadian youth, both second generation and newcomers"; "young Filipina women"	"Artscape Youngplace" shared admin hub		"Youth activate their creativity to explore identity, fostering pride and self-confidence, inspiring and empowering them to realize their full potential"	Performing arts, moving image, design and production, marketing and enterprise	Six-month mentorship and peer program and use of facilities and supplies; 10-week workshop programs	None

(continued)

Organization	City	Date Founded (and Date of Termination, if Relevant)	Turnover 2015 (and over Period)	Number of Students 2015 (and over Period)	Governance Structure	Key Funders 2015
Key Changes (Islington Music Forum Ltd.)	London	1997	2012: £144,100; 2009: £184,047		Charity	Youth Music; ACE; Ministry of Defence Covenant Fund; trusts and foundations—Mencap; corporate donations—Zurich Insurance; alternative education centers, residential care centers, community mental health centers (2009: "therapy contracts")
Kensington Youth Theatre and Employment Skills (KYTES)	Toronto	1983–2003 (still exists as a program of St. Stephens)	Estimated: $300,000			Social services
Lakeshore Arts (Local Arts Service Organization)	Toronto	1993	$431,000	"2,797 children and youth served"	Charity, 1999–	Tritium
Scarborough Arts (Local Arts Service Organization)	Toronto	1978	$467,978		1989–2010 Scarborough Arts Council	Operating: City of Toronto; Ontario Arts Council projects: City of Toronto, Ontario Trillium Foundation, Canadian Heritage, Toronto Foundation, Mitzie Hunter; MPP Donors & Sponsors: Intact Insurance, *The Scarborough Mirror*, Above Ground Art Supplies, Steam Whistle Brewery, Konzelmann Estate Winery (historically: operating grants from the City of Scarborough and Ontario Arts Council)

Type of Student 2015	Property/ Residences 2015 (and over the Period)	Neighborhood (and Character Change over the Period)	Mission 2015	Art Forms 2015	Programs/Mode of Delivery 2015	Accreditation/ Links with Formal Education Providers 2015 (and over the Period)
" 'Hard to reach' patients who may be unresponsive to conventional therapies, non-compliant with medication or experiencing difficulties engaging with other activities or services"	Space within St. Luke's Community Centre	Islington (Index Multiple Deprivation rank of average rank 2015: 13; 2000: 8) (68% White—2011 census)/ London and Winchester/ national	"Promotes well-being and recovery through developing creative, technical and vocational skills and opens pathways to mainstream opportunities in education, training, work experience and employment"	Music	Workshops and courses in hospital and community settings; "open mic" events	None
				Theater, drama	Four months full-time school hours program; mentorship	Some programs with high school accreditation
"People of all ages and backgrounds" "within our neighbourhood"	Rented with city support	Lakeshore	"Committed to improving the availability of arts, cultural and heritage activities within our neighbourhood"	Dance, visual arts	Drop-in classes; community events and exhibitions	None
	Owned 1992–	Scarborough	"We bring artists to the community and community to the arts"	Varied	Professional development workshops; open mic nights; arts education to underserved school communities	None

(*continued*)

Organization	City	Date Founded (and Date of Termination, if Relevant)	Turnover 2015 (and over Period)	Number of Students 2015 (and over Period)	Governance Structure	Key Funders 2015
Urban Arts (Local Arts Service Organization)	Toronto	1988	$786,000		Charity, 2003– (initially "Arts Council for the City of York" and "Arts York")	"Corporate partners include RBC, TELUS, Microsoft Canada and Renewed Computer Technology"
Lyric Hammersmith	London	1888; relaunch 2015	£5,456,007 (2005: £3,537,154)	"Young people undertook 6,430 session attendances" (annual report 2015)	A youth program running as part of a larger theater organization— charity	ACE; Hammersmith & Fulham LA; Mayor of London; trusts and foundations—Reuben Foundation, Esmee Fairborn, Henry Smith Charity, Ideas Tap, Shine Trust, The Ironmongers Company, BBC Children in Need (2005: LB Hammersmith and Fulham, Sure Start Broadway, Association of London Government, ACE, Home Office Refugee Integration Challenge Fund, Paul Hamlyn)

Type of Student 2015	Property/ Residences 2015 (and over the Period)	Neighborhood (and Character Change over the Period)	Mission 2015	Art Forms 2015	Programs/Mode of Delivery 2015	Accreditation/ Links with Formal Education Providers 2015 (and over the Period)
"Under-served, economically disadvantaged and diverse neighborhoods"; "youth"; "females"; "males"	"In May 2002, Arts York, moved to an independent space and launched Y-Arts?, a storefront community arts centre in Weston"	North West Priority Neighbourhood	"Provides for an open, supportive environment for children, youth, and adults in inner-city Toronto with access to free art studio space, instruction and supplies"; "providing opportunities for diverse cultural expression, artistic development, training and employment . . . [and is] an incubator for local arts"; "enhancing neighbourhoods by engaging community through the arts"	Graffiti/mural, theater, yoga, leadership, culinary arts, music, recording studio, spoken word, writing program; dance—partnered with National Ballet and they came in to do workshops; kids also do hip-hop	Multidisciplinary after-school art program; 5 days per week; a number of satellite services including the newly created Girls Mentoring Program at five local schools	None
"Young West Londoners"; "most at risk;" "young people from socially excluded and disadvantaged backgrounds"	Theater studio, film and TV studio, dance studio, cinema, sensory space, recording studio, editing suit, plus the venue proper—in owned Reuben Foundation Wing opened in 2015	Hammersmith & Fulham (Index Multiple Deprivation rank of average rank 2015: 76; 2000: 68) (68% White—2011 census)	"Engages young people . . . in high quality creative learning opportunities to help develop their creative social, personal and economic potential . . . [and] to nurture a new diverse generation of theatre artists, technicians and managers"	Theater	Program for schools and colleges; ongoing after-school classes and workshops including "Young Company" by audition; "targeted activity" by referral; residencies and apprenticeships	None

(continued)

Organization	City	Date Founded (and Date of Termination, if Relevant)	Turnover 2015 (and over Period)	Number of Students 2015 (and over Period)	Governance Structure	Key Funders 2015
The Midi Music Company	London	1995	£256,528 (1995: £78,261; 2005: £396,747)	"336 children participated in instrumental lessons . . . 2,490 young adults . . . received 'one to one' information and guidance" (2015 annual report)	Charity	ACE; Lewisham LA; trusts and foundations—City Bridge Trust, Tom Ap Rhys Pryce Memorial Trust (1995: Lewisham LA, British Council Youth Exchange Centre, Deptford City Challenge; trusts and foundations—Bridge House, Essmee Fairbairn; contract with Lewisham College; 2005: Lewisham LA, ACE, Lottery, Deptford Challenge Trust, Connexions; trusts and foundations—A Glimmer of Hope Trusts, Sound Connections, Sir William Boermans)
Miscellaneous Productions	Vancouver	2000	$281,537 (2005: $267,657)		Charity	Arts Council; Telus

Type of Student 2015	Property/ Residences 2015 (and over the Period)	Neighborhood (and Character Change over the Period)	Mission 2015	Art Forms 2015	Programs/Mode of Delivery 2015	Accreditation/ Links with Formal Education Providers 2015 (and over the Period)
"Children for whom it would not otherwise be available"	Performance hall, rehearsal rooms and recording studio—owned (moved between 2005 and 2015)	Lewisham (Index Multiple Deprivation rank of average rank 2015: 26; 2000: 30) (54% White—2011 census)	"For children and young people to learn how to play instruments, develop music production skills, record their music, develop creative enterprises, explore creative internships, expand their social networks, rehearse, perform and develop themselves as creative entrepreneurs"; (2005: "We're the underground, with some of it breaking through. New talent from Midi is already getting recognition. . . . Right now the creative industries are growing")	Music	Ongoing tuition and workshops in instrument playing, music production, and business; mentoring and creative industry careers advice service; performance events; outreach' projects—a "contract deliverer" for Lewisham and by referral work with young people from "schools, colleges, social services, youth offending schemes, looked after service, youth projects, local housing initiatives, mental health services, employment initiatives and there related agencies" (Historically fixed-term courses for 15- to 19-year-olds NEET etc. with WAC)	None (1995: Foundation in Creative Music and Technology with Lewisham College; 2005: Certificate in Professional Practice in Youth Arts Development in partnership with WAC)
"Culturally and socially representative youth who face multiple barriers"		East Vancouver	"Provides culturally and socially diverse community members with innovative and inspiring performing arts-based opportunities to empower themselves and effect social change and personal transformation"	Performing arts	Workshops; project-based work; mentorship; touring	None

(continued)

Organization	City	Date Founded (and Date of Termination, if Relevant)	Turnover 2015 (and over Period)	Number of Students 2015 (and over Period)	Governance Structure	Key Funders 2015
Newcomer Youth Popular Theatre	Vancouver	2013	$20,000	20	Charity	Mosaic; CLICK; Telus; Coast Capital; Civil Forfeiture Office
NIA	Toronto	2009	$229,400		Charity, 2014–	2009: seed funding from Youth Challenge Fund (United Way)
Oasis Skateboard Factory	Toronto	2007		25 per semester	One program in the Oasis Alternative Secondary School	Toronto District School Board (TDSB); numerous corporate sponsors

Type of Student 2015	Property/ Residences 2015 (and over the Period)	Neighborhood (and Character Change over the Period)	Mission 2015	Art Forms 2015	Programs/Mode of Delivery 2015	Accreditation/ Links with Formal Education Providers 2015 (and over the Period)
Immigrant or refugee youth aged 14–24 years		Vancouver	"A space for youth to share their issues and seek positive solutions and at the same time, increases community awareness on the challenges faced by newcomer youth"	Theater	Performance-based learning	None
"Suffering discrimination, particularly from racial discrimination, or poverty"; "With a talent or passion for art"	Renting below market rate from the city in a former Toronto Public Health building	Throughout the city	"Nia is a Kiswahili term meaning "purpose"; "The organization focuses on supporting young people in finding their purpose"; "We provide programming and services to engage people artistically, emotionally, spiritually, and intellectually in order to support the development of healthy identities and positive life choices"; "In addition to delivering culturally specific programming, Nia Centre showcases and promotes arts from an African Diasporic perspective in a way that engages inter-generational artists and the general population"	"Media arts," "digital arts," "drumming," "photography"; special programs available in "arts and business" and "carnival arts"	Workshops; mentorship; annual concerts/ exhibitions; programming in schools and community settings	None
"Youth living on the margins"	Owned and managed by TDSB—one of Oasis Alternative Schools started in the TDSB	Downtown	"Re-engagement"	Design and production	Skateboard Factory "courses with a skateboard and street art focus where students earn credits by operating a socially responsible entrepreneurial business"	High school diploma

(continued)

Organization	City	Date Founded (and Date of Termination, if Relevant)	Turnover 2015 (and over Period)	Number of Students 2015 (and over Period)	Governance Structure	Key Funders 2015
Ovalhouse	London	1937	£1,029,957 (1995: £429,223; 2005: £778,385)		A youth program running as part of a larger theater organization—charity	ACE, Lambeth LA; trusts and foundations (1995: Lambeth LA, London Councils; 2005: Lambeth LA, ACE, trusts and foundations—Paul Hamlyn)
Paddington Arts	London	1983	£241,140 (1995: £91,254; 2005: £310,847)	"2429 total of young people worked with"; "65 average number of individuals attending workshops per week"	Charity	Westminster LA, ACE, Heritage Lottery Fund; trusts and foundations—London Youth (1995: Westminster LA, ACE, trust and foundations—Rank Foundation, John Lyon's Charity; 2005: Westminster LA, Single Regeneration Budget, ACE, trusts and foundations—Rank Foundation, John Lyon's Charity, Bridge House Trust, Children's Fund)
The Remix Project	Toronto	1999				

Type of Student 2015	Property/ Residences 2015 (and over the Period)	Neighborhood (and Character Change over the Period)	Mission 2015	Art Forms 2015	Programs/Mode of Delivery 2015	Accreditation/ Links with Formal Education Providers 2015 (and over the Period)
"From the hardest to reach to those that are hard to keep away" (Historically "refugees or asylum seekers" "excluded for school" unemployed)	Two theater spaces, rehearsal studios, workshops spaces, café bar—owned and extended several times over life span. Will be moving to brand new purpose-built venue in Brixton center funded by Lambeth LA, ACE, and fundraising	Lambeth (Index Multiple Deprivation rank of average rank 2015: 22; 2000: 21) (57% White—2011 census)	"Provid[es] a space where artists can develop their creative practice, audiences can encounter new work and see the beginnings of new talent, and young people can use the arts to look at their lives, and develop their creativity and skills"	Theater	Ongoing youth theaters; youth arts festival; projects in collaboration with other organizations; mentorship and training schemes	None
"[Those who] enjoy dance, drama, singing, playing steel pan or even participating in the Notting Hill carnival" (2005: "socially excluded groups such as young offenders, young disabled and young unemployed")	Main hall, dance studio, rehearsal room, digital newsroom—bought from the LA in 1990 with Lottery money (initially taking place in church hall)	Westminster (2015: Index Multiple Deprivation rank of average rank: 43; 2000: 141) (62% White—2011 census)	"Provide[s] a safe space for children and young people to take part in creative activities; learn new skills; make new friends; broaden their horizons; and help them to find their place in the world"	Performing arts, media, carnival	Ongoing performing arts classes; carnival season work; annual trip to Paddington Farm; video and journalism projects	None (2005: experimented with "our first accredited learning programme in Community Dance")

(continued)

Organization	City	Date Founded (and Date of Termination, if Relevant)	Turnover 2015 (and over Period)	Number of Students 2015 (and over Period)	Governance Structure	Key Funders 2015
Raw Material Music and Media	London	1993	£579,546 (2005: £310,550)	"Over 500 people" (annual report 2015)	Charity	ACE, Lambeth LA, trusts and foundations—Comic Relief, People's Health Trust, Lloyds Foundation Trust, Goldsmiths Company, Garfield Weston Foundation (2005: ACE, London Development Agency, trusts and foundations—John Lyon's Charity)
Reel2Real	Vancouver	1998	$313,849 (2012: $243,174; 2005: $154,842)	2005: 741 students (animating kids final report)	Charity	Government; corporate; foundations
Reel Youth	Vancouver	2005		4,000	Charity	Government; fee for service; foundations

Type of Student 2015	Property/ Residences 2015 (and over the Period)	Neighborhood (and Character Change over the Period)	Mission 2015	Art Forms 2015	Programs/Mode of Delivery 2015	Accreditation/ Links with Formal Education Providers 2015 (and over the Period)
"We work in mental health in hospitals and the community with children, young people and adults, with CAMHS (Children and Adolescent Mental Health Services), in SEND (Special Educational Needs and Disabilities), within youth offending and with children and young people in challenging circumstances"	"Three recording studios, a live room and rehearsal space, a music technology suite with fifteen workstations, film and photography resources, a range of musical instruments, drums, amplifiers and sound systems and a small performance space with stage lighting and PA system"	Lambeth (Index Multiple Deprivation rank of average rank 2015: 22; 2000: 21) (57% White— 2011 census)	"Improve[s] the lives of young people and their economic position, their opportunities, progression and development, including mental and physical health issues"	Music and media	Ongoing after-school classes in instruments, voice, and production; artist development mentorship; projects in collaboration with health and education service	Assessment and Qualifications Alliance qualification
"Gender-neutral and safe for all students and patrons"		Vancouver; sometimes provincial	"[S]how[s] the best in culturally diverse, authentic programming for youth"	Film	Project-based work; film festival; youth jury; school partnerships	None
"Youth 19 years and under"		National	"Create[s] positive change in young people's lives through technical skill building, leadership training, creative collaboration with peers and mentors, and increased connection to community resources"	Film	Project-based work; film festival; youth jury; school partnerships	None

(continued)

Organization	City	Date Founded (and Date of Termination, if Relevant)	Turnover 2015 (and over Period)	Number of Students 2015 (and over Period)	Governance Structure	Key Funders 2015
Regent Park Focus Youth Media Centre	Toronto	1990		More than 5,000 young people have participated in the past 15 years (website)	Charity, 1993 (then gave it up to become part of a Focus Community)	
RISE (Reaching Intelligent Souls Everywhere) Edutainment	Toronto	2012				
Rising Tide	London	2001	£66,400 (2005: £78,677; 2004: £226,187)	"This year we have delivered programmes to 1000 people. . . . We have also supported more than 20 young people towards developing a career within the music industry" (annual report, 2015)	Charity	Hackney LA; trusts and foundations— Damilola Taylor Trust

Type of Student 2015	Property/ Residences 2015 (and over the Period)	Neighborhood (and Character Change over the Period)	Mission 2015	Art Forms 2015	Programs/Mode of Delivery 2015	Accreditation/ Links with Formal Education Providers 2015 (and over the Period)
"High risk youth," "Young women"	Arts center	Regent Park community	"A community learning centre for new media, digital arts, and radio & television broadcasting. We provide a community facility dedicated to the training and mentorship of young people and the engagement of community members of all ages"	Radio, TV, magazine, photography, music, new media word, music, journalism, events	"A variety of free multi-media programs all year round to youth. Tackling social justice issues through the use of audio, video and new media technology. The youth have the opportunity to gain experience in many different types of broadcasting equipment, software and journalistic practices"; mentorship	None
"A community led by youth, comprised of artists, activists, free-thinkers and revolutionaries" overwhelmingly youth of color	Hosted in community center	Scarborough	"Help[s] to create a safe and welcoming platform for self-expression and healing through the performance arts"	Spoken word, events	Weekly open mic	None
"Young people with a passion for making music"; "some of London's most deprived young people and communities"	Rehearsal rooms and recording studio—owned	Hackney (Index Multiple Deprivation rank of average rank 2015: 2; 2000: 2) (55% White—2011 census)	"Rising Tide's ability to help turn people's lives around by raising aspirations, attainment and a self confidence is second to none, as the place where many young people grow up into upstanding members of their communities, holding down steady jobs, or even becoming professionals within the media industry." "A music-based creative hub for young people with a passion for making music . . . supporting young artists to become household names"	Music	"Open door policy—with a Capitalise Animating Kids approach to offering services"; music tutoring and mentoring, "industry specific opportunities"; project-based work on estates; partnerships with Hackney Museum, Hackney Creative Quarter	None

(continued)

Organization	City	Date Founded (and Date of Termination, if Relevant)	Turnover 2015 (and over Period)	Number of Students 2015 (and over Period)	Governance Structure	Key Funders 2015
Roundhouse Studios	London	2005	£11,257,174 (2005: £7,569,109)	"This year we worked with 3,323 young people" (2015 report)	A youth program and performing arts and concert venue created together to be symbiotic—charity	ACE, Youth Music, trusts and foundations—Paul Hamlin, Esme Fairbairn, The Andrew Lloyd Webber Foundation, The Monument Trust, Garfield Weston Foundation, John Lyon's Charity, Amy Winehouse Foundation; corporate donors—Bloomberg (2005: ACE, Camden LA, trusts and foundations—Paul Hamlyn/founded with money from The Normal Trust, DfE, donations)
Saint James Music Academy	Vancouver	2007	$868,863 (2012: $280,583)	2015: 190 students enrolled; 2007: 90 students (website)	Charity	Government; corporate; foundations
Sarah McLachlan School of Music	Vancouver	2002	2012: $1,111,292; 2015: $1,352,552		Charity	Fundraising
Second Wave Youth Arts	London	1982	£128,909 (1995: £101,112; 2005: £215,144)		Charity	Lewisham LA, Home Office (Prevent), MOPAC, National Lottery; trusts and foundations—Esme Fairbairn, BBC Children in Need (1995: Lewisham LA, Deplored Youth Forum, Arts Council London, City Challenge; 2005: Lewisham LA, Connexions, Arts Council England, trusts and foundations—Esme Fairbairn, Millennium Volunteers Fund)

Type of Student 2015	Property/ Residences 2015 (and over the Period)	Neighborhood (and Character Change over the Period)	Mission 2015	Art Forms 2015	Programs/Mode of Delivery 2015	Accreditation/ Links with Formal Education Providers 2015 (and over the Period)
"No matter what their background"; "A diverse community of young creatives"	Purpose-built band rehearsal rooms, recording studio, media production suites, TV studio, plus the venue proper—owned since founding	Camden (Index Multiple Deprivation rank of average rank 2015: 69; 2000: 56) (66% White—2011 census)	"Offer[s] . . . over 3,000 young people exceptional creative opportunities enabling them to build skills for employment and personal development"	Performing arts and media	Ongoing drop-in sessions, term-length weekly workshops and one-off masterclasses; "outreach" work with schools, pupil referral units and community groups; intensive courses for NEETs	None
Inner city youth		Downtown Eastside	"Inspire[s] Vancouver's inner city youth to bring social transformation through the power and joy of music"	Music	After-school and community programming; school workshops; concerts	None
Underserved and at-risk youth (website)		Vancouver, Surrey, Edmonton	"Provide[s] high quality music programming in a safe, nurturing environment to children, youth and seniors that face barriers in their access to music education"	Music	After-school and community programming	None
"From BME communities"; "local young women"	Studio and rehearsal space in Deptford Methodist Mission	Lewisham (Index Multiple Deprivation rank of average rank 2015: 26; 2000: 30) (54% White—2011 census)	"Enables youth participation in local decision-making, supports youth-led initiatives in their neighbourhoods, strengthens the well-being of young people, and helps them to make informed choices about their lives"; "support young people to produce and perform work relevant to their lives and experiences"	Performing arts, writing	Ongoing evening and weekend performing arts workshops; forums and debates; leadership traineeships; projects in collaboration with schools, colleges, and community organizations	None

(continued)

Organization	City	Date Founded (and Date of Termination, if Relevant)	Turnover 2015 (and over Period)	Number of Students 2015 (and over Period)	Governance Structure	Key Funders 2015
SKETCH	Toronto	1990	$1,996,454	600	Not for profit—2001; charity, 2003–	Ontario Arts Council; Ontario Trilium Foundation; private foundations (first grant from the Department of Health in 1994)
Some Assembly Arts Society	Vancouver	1995	2015: $106,153 (2014: $113,577)	More than 2,500 (website)	Charity	Government; corporate; foundations
South Asian Arts	Vancouver	2005	2015: $25,698		Nonprofit organization	Fee for service; government funding
Streetrich Hiphop	Vancouver	2012	2015: $6,000	300	Nonprofit organization	City of Surrey; City of Vancouver; Vancouver Foundation; TD Bank; BC Arts Council
Studio 3 Arts	London	1988	£496,746 (1997: £84,933; 2005: £238,590)	"In 2014/15, we delivered more than 47 projects to an audience of over 11,000 people"	A youth program running as part of a larger theater organization—charity	ACE, Barking and Dagenham LA, Havering LA. trusts and foundations—Children In Need, Taylor Wimpey (2005: ACE, Barking and Dagenham LA, Havering LA, Connexions, Bridge House Estates)

Type of Student 2015	Property/ Residences 2015 (and over the Period)	Neighborhood (and Character Change over the Period)	Mission 2015	Art Forms 2015	Programs/Mode of Delivery 2015	Accreditation/ Links with Formal Education Providers 2015 (and over the Period)
"Living street involved, homeless or otherwise on the margins"; "youth navigating adversity"	Studio space in ArtScape Youngplace since 2012 (several previous spaces)		"Creates opportunities for young people . . . to experience the transformative power of the arts; to build leadership and economic self-sufficiency in the arts; and to cultivate social and environmental change through the arts"	Visual arts	"Open studio"; more structured "drug project"	None
Diverse youth (website)		Vancouver	"Creates employment, increases the well-being of youth and advances education by providing mentorship and workshops for youth on topics related to performing arts, mental health and addiction"	Theater	Production based	None
"Professional and amateur artists"		Vancouver, Surrey	"Build[s] artistic forums that act as a platform for building knowledge of South Asian culture"	Performing arts	Ongoing classes; performing arts festival; workshops; school partnerships	Credits for high school diploma
"In this place youth from all walks of life come together as equal participants" (old website)		Vancouver, Surrey	"Connects individuals through the language of Hip Hop, giving marginalized youth a unique voice to share their stories, breaking stereotypes, and contributing to a global community of change"	Performing and visual arts		None
"Communities"; "the public"; "local people"; "young people"	Theater, recording studios, gardens— owned	Barking and Dagenham (Index Multiple Deprivation rank of average rank 2015: 3; 2000: 24) (58% White— 2011 census)	"Create[s] brilliant, challenging and relevant work that acknowledges and responds to the barriers that prevent arts participation"	Theater, music and spoken word, media	Ongoing after-school classes; "professional development" training; open mic and emerging artist platforms	"Industry-standard training in performing arts and professional practice"

(continued)

Organization	City	Date Founded (and Date of Termination, if Relevant)	Turnover 2015 (and over Period)	Number of Students 2015 (and over Period)	Governance Structure	Key Funders 2015
Talk to Youth Lately	Toronto		35,288	25 young people plus hundreds of high school and university student audiences and workshops	Previously Ministry of Health Promotion	
The AM& (Artists Mentoring Youth) Project	Toronto	2005	$67,000 (2010: $30,000)			Ontario Arts Council (first Ontario Arts Council Project Grant was $8,000 in 2005)

Type of Student 2015	Property/ Residences 2015 (and over the Period)	Neighborhood (and Character Change over the Period)	Mission 2015	Art Forms 2015	Programs/Mode of Delivery 2015	Accreditation/ Links with Formal Education Providers 2015 (and over the Period)
	Rented publicly	Landsdown and Bloor/ Parkdale	Anti-stigma	Visual arts, circus arts	"Providing performances in public places and educational institutions— to educate and increase the public's understanding of circus—to provide instructional seminars on topics related to the performing and visual arts—to produce performing arts festivals for the purposes of educating artists through participation in such festivals and related workshops"; circus arts, food for participants, youth employment (twelve 14- to 17-year-olds trained per year), mental health focus— create circus work for raising issues about mental health	None
"Young women"; in 2015, the program added "nonbinary youth"	In kind from Jumblies Theatre	Currently downtown	"Aims to nurture the confidence and identity of participating young women by increasing their cultural vocabulary and engaging them in activities of healthy, creative self-expression"	Performing arts	The collective creation of theatre; "group, and one-to-one training sessions to further artistic and leadership development"; meals and transportation; performance opportunities; partnerships with other organizations	None

(continued)

Organization	City	Date Founded (and Date of Termination, if Relevant)	Turnover 2015 (and over Period)	Number of Students 2015 (and over Period)	Governance Structure	Key Funders 2015
The Cinematheque	Vancouver	1984	1995: $347,694; 2005: $890,728; 2015: $918,019	+3,500	Charity	Government
The Remix Project	Toronto	1999	$765,718	"Over 400 youth apply to Remix each semester with only 45 spots available in the three academies"	Charity, 2009– (Inner City Visions–2006)	TD Bank, Sennheiser, Cineplex, the RBC Foundation, The Government of Ontario, the Ontario Arts Council, City of Toronto
The Video College	London	1994	£64,085 (1995: £169,601; 2005: £303,756)	"Over 200 young people" (2005 annual report)	Charity	Kensington & Chelsea LA; British Film Institute; Indie Training Fund: "We continue to be affected by cutbacks and the BFI's main focus on young people viewing rather than making films" (1995: Kensington & Chelsea LA, City Challenge, trusts and foundations—City Parochial Foundation, Henry Smith's Charity, Foundation for Sports and the Arts, Esmee Fairbairn; 2005: Holborn SRB, Paddington Development Trusts, Neighbourhood Renewal Fund, Film London, European Social Fund, trusts and foundations—Campden Charities, Tudor Trusts, Kensington Housing Trust, Headly Trust)

Type of Student 2015	Property/ Residences 2015 (and over the Period)	Neighborhood (and Character Change over the Period)	Mission 2015	Art Forms 2015	Programs/Mode of Delivery 2015	Accreditation/ Links with Formal Education Providers 2015 (and over the Period)
Youth, young audiences		Vancouver	"Foster[s] a critical understanding of the impact of visual media in the world around us, and an appreciation for the exciting art of filmmaking"	Media	After-school and community programming	None
"Young people from disadvantaged, marginalized and under served communities"; "youth who are trying to enter into the creative industries or further their formal education"; "disengaged by the system available to them"			"Top-notch alternative, creative, educational programs, facilitators and facilities. Our mission is to help refine the raw talents of young people in order to help them find success as participants define it and on their own terms"; "The Remix Project's vision is to become an internationally recognized destination for recruiters from post-secondary institutions and corporations looking for fresh and exciting young talent and leaders"	Started with the four elements of hip hop: turntables, graffiti, rap battles, and breakdance competitions under the name ICV; visual arts focus incorporated in 2002; business focus in 2001 onwards	Creative Arts Program, Recording Arts Program, Business Arts Program, Young Entrepreneur Business Incubator Program, performance opportunities	Some programs with high school accreditation
"Disadvantaged young people"; "those traditionally under-represented in the media"	Space in Westway Trust building (1995: "minuscule office by the Wornington Green Estate"—set up by local residents association)	Kensington & Chelsea (Index Multiple Deprivation rank of average rank 2015: 99 2000: 202) (71% White—2011 census)	"Provides production facilities and training in all areas of Arts and Media for disadvantaged young people"	Film	Ongoing after-school classes; holiday program; vocational training courses	'Industry standard' training (2005: one of only five Industry Training Providers acknowledged by Skillset—Level 1 LOCN Introduction to video course, NVQ Level 2 City and Guilds Television and Media Competences, Level 2 & 3 LOCN Combined Production Course in Specialist Skills)

(continued)

Organization	City	Date Founded (and Date of Termination, if Relevant)	Turnover 2015 (and over Period)	Number of Students 2015 (and over Period)	Governance Structure	Key Funders 2015
Unity Charity	Toronto	2004	$1,220,060	200,896 youth reached between 2012 and 2016	Charity, 2007–	Laidlaw Foundation; corporate sponsors—many, including Canadian Heritage, Royal Bank, CIBC, Great West Life, London Life, Canada Life, TD Bank, City of Toronto, AGO, ArtStarts, Toronto Public Health, Tangerine, Jays
Vibe Arts	Toronto	1995	$1,170,474		Nonprofit (formally Arts for Children of Toronto)	Community partners
WAC Arts (WAC Performing Arts Media College)	London	1978	£1,620,763 (1995: £1,013,464; 2005: £2,131,213)	"In 2014/15 . . . enriching the lives of 1,000 young people throughout the year"; 2005–2015: 800	Charity	Camden LA, European Social Fund, trusts and foundations—BBC Children in Need, City Bridge Trust, John Lyon's Charity, The Sobell Foundation, Tuxien Foundation, U3A in London; donations and fundraising (1995: Camden LA, London Boroughs Grants Scheme, Arts Council London; 2005: Camden LA, Sure Start, Association of London Government, London Development Agency, ACE, European Social Fund, trusts and foundations—Esmee Fairbairn, John Lyon's Charity, City Parochial Foundation)

Type of Student 2015	Property/ Residences 2015 (and over the Period)	Neighborhood (and Character Change over the Period)	Mission 2015	Art Forms 2015	Programs/Mode of Delivery 2015	Accreditation/ Links with Formal Education Providers 2015 (and over the Period)
			To use hip hop to create healthier communities; "to promote artistic expression containing a message of non-violence and tolerance, positive forms of self-expression, and their impact on the community"	Spoken word, music, dance	After-school and community programming; school workshops and assemblies; festivals	None
"Children and youth in under-resourced communities"; "marginalized youth"; "emerging artists"		"Neighbour-hood Improvement Areas"	"Works collaboratively . . . to innovate, build skills and resiliency, and lead social change http://zizics.com/ profile/Preid through arts education programming"	Multi—performing arts, writing, visual arts, cultural heritage arts	"Multi-disciplinary arts programs, which take place directly in shelters, public housing, libraries, schools, parks, hospitals, detention and community centres. Every VIBE program features youth mentorship, leadership, learning and employment opportunities"; micro-grants	None
"Talented"; "marginalised"; "experiencing exceptional hardship and challenges"	Hampstead Town Hall: theater, dance studios, music rooms, recording studio, sensory pod—owned since 1999 (originally hosted in a building run by Intermedia in the same area)	Camden (Index Multiple Deprivation rank of average rank 2015: 69; 2000: 56) (66% White—2011 census)	"A place where diverse talent, often from challenging backgrounds, can be safely nurtured though the highest quality performing arts and media education"; "outstanding levels of art and media training . . . for those wanting a career in the arts"	Performing arts and media	Ongoing classes for "junior" 6- to 14-year-old and "senior" 14- and 15-year-old young people and young people with disabilities/ learning difficulties; Holiday projects; (historically fixed-period intensive courses for young people by referral); higher education courses	Diploma in Professional Music Theatre; in 2014, WAC opened the first alternative provision free school—funded by central government, offering formal education qualifications, etc. (2005: OCN Levels 1–3 qualifications in Music Technology; Foundation Degree/Diploma in Performing Arts accredited by Trinity)

(continued)

Organization	City	Date Founded (and Date of Termination, if Relevant)	Turnover 2015 (and over Period)	Number of Students 2015 (and over Period)	Governance Structure	Key Funders 2015
Youth in 57 Minutes	Vancouver	2004			Past Project	Funded by City of Vancouver in the past
Young People's Press	Toronto	1997–2004	Roughly 120,000–150,000	300–400 writers; 600–1,200 workshop recipients	Part of Canadian Centre for Social Justice	
Young Urban Arts Foundation	London	2009	£140,672	"By 2021 we will empower over 15,000 young people per year"	Charity	LAs; housing associations; trusts and foundations

ACE, Arts Council England; BAME, Black, Asian, and minority ethnic; LA, local authority: NEET, not in education, employment, or training; NVQ, National Vocational Qualification; TDSB, Toronto District School Board; WAC, Weekend Arts College.

* Unattributed quotations are taken from internal and frequently undated paper-based documents (promotional material, unpublished flyers etc.) shared by the organizations.

Type of Student 2015	Property/ Residences 2015 (and over the Period)	Neighborhood (and Character Change over the Period)	Mission 2015	Art Forms 2015	Programs/Mode of Delivery 2015	Accreditation/ Links with Formal Education Providers 2015 (and over the Period)
"Dedicated to representing young adults and addressing issues not covered by mainstream media"		Vancouver	"Allow[s] youth to get actively involved in their community, and also provide[s] a means to let their peers stay informed on issues and local events"	Broadcasting and music	Radio show	None
Targeted outreach to historically disadvantaged communities, particularly racialized ones; but also workshops in secondary schools for any/all student			To give young people aged 14–24 years a voice in the mainstream media	Journalism		None
"Vulnerable and disadvantaged young people"	Outreach media business- owned since founding	London	"Helps vulnerable and disadvantaged young people . . . learn new skills, but also builds confidence, self-esteem and self-worth—with many going on to experience . . . further training"	Music	One-off workshops and longer term programs in partnership with other organizations/ bodies	None

NOTES

Chapter 1

1. Throughout the book we refer to costs in Canadian dollars and pounds sterling. Because of the difficulty of translating currency conversion rates historically, we have left all costs in the format where we found them in their original currencies.

Chapter 2

1. See, for example, https://criminalizingdissent.wordpress.com/2012/11/05/yonge-street-riot-1992; https://www.thecanadianencyclopedia.ca/en/article/murder-of-reena-virk; https://localwiki.org/toronto/Summer_of_The_Gun; https://www.bbc.co.uk/news/uk-england-london-36977810.

2. https://www.gov.uk/government/organisations/companies-house.

3. https://apps.cra-arc.gc.ca/ebci/hacc/srch/pub/dsplyBscSrch.

Chapter 3

1. For a definition of a LASO, see https://www.toronto.ca/services-payments/grants-incentives-rebates/arts-culture-grants.

2. Dates in parentheses after organizations' names refer to the year they were established.

3. Please note, the authors drew from the public document, *The Remix Project: A Brief History*, to support the following account. This document is available at https://theremix project.com/

Chapter 4

1. https://vimeo.com/34556338.

Chapter 5

1. Education is managed differently in Scotland and Northern Ireland and Wales.

2. The end of Thatcherism under John Major; the period of New Labour, 1997–2010, under Tony Blair and Gordon Brown; and the Conservative-led coalition, 2010–2015, led by David Cameron.

3. It is worth noting the choice of the term "free schools": " 'Free schools' have a strong anarchist and libertarian history—from freethinking Jewish schools at the end of the nineteenth century to London's infamous White Lion Free School in the 1970s. . . . From the working-class autodidactic traditions of the eighteenth and nineteenth centuries . . . to the

radical socialist and feminist educational cultures at the turn of the century . . . to the aspirational and radical cultures of migrant communities . . ., alternative schooling has long played a part in Britain's education system" (Gerrard, 2014, pp. 878–879).

4. English Baccalaureate, the informal name for the current arrangement of examination subjects to be taken at age 16 years, at the time of writing.

Chapter 6

1. Despite historical and ongoing state-sanctioned social, physical, economic, and cultural violence (Razack, 2002; A. Smith, 2005), many Indigenous communities in Canada have preserved their worldviews and have demonstrated ongoing resilience in the face of injustice and inequality (Flicker et al., 2014, p. 17).

2. Ovalhouse is now Brixton House (https://brixtonhouse.co.uk/our-story/from-ovalhouse-to-brixton-house).

Chapter 8

1. A prestigious leadership development award aimed at capacity-building professionalized management in the arts, not dissimilar to Alberta's Future Leaders (https://www.affta.ab.ca/funding/special-programs/alberta-future-leaders) or Mentorship and Youth Engagement, a new initiative in British Columbia (https://bctouring.org/programs-services/mye).

2. W. M. Keck Foundation (https://www.wmkeck.org/grant-programs/grant-progr ams).

Chapter 9

1. https://assets.publishing.service.gov.uk/government/uploads/system/uploads/atta chment_data/file/78979/building-big-society_0.pdf.

Chapter 10

1. And as a coda to this thread of the discussion, we note that the effects of social isolation as a consequence of the COVID-19 pandemic lockdown in 2020 and 2021 have already raised questions about the need to sustain forms of provision for young people and, indeed, the realization that it may be signaling an end to the forms and traditions described in the preceding chapters (see Hill, 2021).

2. https://www.bighart.org/evidence/evaluation-essay.

REFERENCES

Adler, J. (2011, June 24). SKETCH art studio encourages creative potential of street youth. *SamaritanMag.* https://www.samaritanmag.com/sketch-art-studio-encourages-creat ive-potential-street-youth

Alastair, S., & Brian, H. (2019). Institutional amnesia and public policy. *Journal of European Public Policy, 26*(10), 1521–1539. https://doi.org/10.1080/13501763.2018.1535612

Amin, A. (2014). Lively infrastructure. *Theory, Culture & Society, 31*(7–8), 137–161.

Amsler, S. S. (2015). *The education of radical democracy.* Routledge.

Andris, C., Liu, X., Mitchell, J., O'Dwyer, J., & van Cleve, J. (2021). Threads across the urban fabric: Youth mentorship relationships as neighborhood bridges. *Journal of Urban Affairs, 43*(1), 77–92. https://doi.org/10.1080/07352166.2019.1662726

Arts Education Partnership. (1999). *Champions of change: The impact of the arts on learning.* Arts Education Partnership & Presidents Committee on Arts and Humanities.

Arvast, A. (2008). The new CAAT: (Dis)illusions of freedom and the New College Charter in Ontario. *Canadian Journal of Higher Education, 38*(1), 105–121.

Baars, S., Bernardes, E., Elwick, A., Malortie, A., McAleavy, T., Mcinerney, L., Menzies, L., & Riggall, A. (2014). *Lessons from London schools: Investigating the success.* CfBT Education Trust.

Baker, D. (2014). *The schooled society: The educational transformation of global culture.* Stanford University Press.

Baker, S., & Edwards, R. (2012). How many qualitative interviews is enough? [Review paper]. National Centre for Research Methods.

Baldridge, B. J. (2019). *Reclaiming community: Race and the uncertain future of youth work.* Stanford University Press.

Ball, S. (2012). The reluctant state and the beginning of the end of state education. *Journal of Educational Administration and History, 442,* 89–103.

Barker, D. K. (2012). Querying the paradox of caring labor. *Rethinking Marxism, 24*(4), 574– 591. https://doi.org/10.1080/08935696.2012.711065

Barker, J., Kauanui, J. K., Denetdale, J., Goeman, M., Perea, J. B., Rifkin, M., Byrd, J. A., & Nelson, M. K. (2017). *Critically sovereign: Indigenous gender, sexuality, and feminist studies.* Duke University Press.

Barker, M. (2013). *The innovators: Interview with Craig Morrison and Laura Hortie, Oasis Skateboard Factory.* https://michaelbarker.ca/notes-from-the-field-alternative-educat ion/fieldwork-talking-with-teachers-in-alternative-schools/oasis-skateboard-factory

Batacharya, S. (2000). *Racism, "girl violence" and the murder of Reena Virk* [Master's thesis]. University of Toronto. https://tspace.library.utoronto.ca/bitstream/1807/13803/1/ MQ49780.pdf

Beck, U. (1992). *Risk society: Towards a new modernity* (M. Ritter, Trans.). SAGE.

Becko, L. (2012). *Mapping non-formal music provision and social need in London*. Sound Connections.

Bekerman, Z., Burbules, N. C., Keller, D. S., & Silberman-Keller, D. (2005). *Learning in places: The informal education reader*. Lang.

Belfield, C., Crawford, C., & Sibieta, L. (2017). *Long-run comparisons of spending per pupil across different stages of education*. Institute for Fiscal Studies.

Bennett, A. (2017). Youth, music and DIY careers. *Cultural Sociology, 12*(2), 133–139.

Berliner, L. S. (2018). *Producing queer youth: The paradox of digital media empowerment*. Routledge.

Bianchini, F. (1987). GLC RIP: Cultural policies in London 1981–1986. *New Formations, 1*.

BMG Research. (2015). *Investigating the school improvement needs and practices of London primary and secondary schools*. Greater London Authority.

Boal, A. (2008). *Theatre of the oppressed* (New ed.). Pluto.

Boudreau, J., Keil, R., & Young, D. (2009). *Changing Toronto: Governing urban neoliberalism*. University of Toronto Press.

Bourdieu, P. (1990). *The logic of practice*. Polity.

Bourdieu, P. (1993). *The field of cultural production: Essays on art and literature*. Polity.

Bourriaud, N. (2002). *Relational aesthetics*. Les Presses du Réel.

Boye, S. (2016). *Looking for social dance in Toronto's Black population at mid-century: A historiography* [Dissertation]. University of Toronto.

Bray, M. (2009). *Confronting the shadow education system: What government policies for what private tutoring?* United Nations Educational, Scientific and Cultural Organization/ International Institute for Educational Planning.

Brine, J. (2002). *European Social Fund and the EU: Flexibility, growth, stability*. Sheffield.

British Columbia Arts Council. (2021). *Program guidelines 2020/21*. www.bcartscouncil.ca/app/ uploads/sites/508/2021/02/FY2021-Community-Arts-Festivals-REVISED-FINAL.pdf

Broom, C. A. (2016). Power, politics, democracy and reform: A historical review of curriculum reform, academia and government in British Columbia, Canada, 1920 to 2000. *Journal of Curriculum Studies, 48*(5), 711–727. www.tandfonline.com/doi/abs/10.1080/ 00220272.2015.1069402

Brough, M. (2020). *Youth power in precarious times*. Duke University Press.

Brown, P., Lauder, H., & Ashton, D. (2011). *The global auction: The broken promises of education, jobs, and incomes*. Oxford University Press.

Brown, S., Delve, W., Gustafsson, T., Peer, A., Pichette, J., Sky, M., Chorzepa, C., & Costa, S. (2017). LGBTQ education timeline. Elementary Teachers Federation of Ontario and Canadian and Lesbian Archives. www.etfo.ca/socialjusticeunion/2slgbtq/lgbtq-educat ion-timeline

Browne, G. (2003). Integrated service delivery: More effective and less expensive. *Ideas That Matter, 2*(3). www.ideasthatmatter.com/quarterly/itm-2-3/vol2no3.pdf

Brunet-Jailly, E. (2008). Vancouver: The sustainable city. *Journal of Urban Affairs, 30*(4), 375–388.

Buckingham, D., Grahame, J., & Sefton-Green, J. (1995). *Making media: Learning from media production*. English & Media Centre.

Buckingham, D., & Jones, K. (2001). New Labour's cultural turn: Some tensions in contemporary educational and cultural policy. *Journal of Education Policy, 16*(1), 1–14.

Bukhari, S. N. (2019). Ethnic media as alternative media for South Asians in Metro Vancouver, Canada: Creating knowledge, engagement, civic and political awareness. *Journal of Alternative and Community Media, 4*(3), 86–98.

Burns Owens Partnership & Stanley, D. (2004). *Supporting talent into enterprise.* BOP Consulting.

Butcher, M., & Dickens, L. (2016). Spatial dislocation and affective displacement: Youth perspectives on gentrification in London. *International Journal of Urban and Regional Research, 40*(4), 800–816.

Cabinet Office, Strategy Unit. (2002). Private action, public benefit: A review of charities and the wider not-for-profit sector. https://philea.issuelab.org/resource/private-act ion-public-benefit-a-review-of-charities-and-the-wider-non-profit-sector-strategy-unit-report-september-2002.html

Campbell, M. (2013). *Out of the basement.* McGill-Queen's University Press.

Campbell, M. (2019). From youth engagement to creative industries incubators: Models of working with youth in community arts settings. *Review of Education, Pedagogy, and Cultural Studies, 41*(3), 164–192. https://doi.org/10.1080/10714413.2019.1685854

Canada Council for the Arts. (2007). *The evolution of the Canada Council's support for the arts.*

Care Collective. (2020). *The care manifesto: The politics of interdependence.* Verso.

Chatterton, P., & Hollands, R. (2002). Theorizing urban playscapes: Producing, regulating and consuming youthful nightlife city spaces. *Urban Studies, 39*(1), 95–116.

Chawla, L. (Ed.). (2002). *Growing up in an urbanising world.* Earthscan.

Christensen, P., & O'Brien, M. (2003). Children in the city: Introducing new paradigms. In P. Christensen & M. O'Brien (Eds.), *Children in the city: Home, neighbourhood and community* (pp. 1–12). RoutledgeFalmer.

Christie, S. (2020). Youth as subjects and agents of artistic research: A comparison of youth engagement models. *Theatre Research in Canada, 41*(2), 308–312.

City of Toronto Archives. (1940). *University settlement music school minutes* (Series 619, Subseries 2, File 23).

Coles, A. (2007, November). Focus on youth: Canadian youth arts programming and policy. In Focus. Canadian Cultural Observatory.

Cornforth, C. (2012). Nonprofit governance research: Limitations of the focus on boards and suggestions for new directions. *Non-Profit and Volunteer Sector Quarterly, 41*(6), 1116–1135.

Crath, R. (2017). Governing youth as an aesthetic and spatial practice. *Urban Studies, 54*(5), 1263–1279.

Crehan, K. (2011). *Community art: An anthropological perspective.* Berg.

Creigh-Tyte, S., & Gallimore, J. (2000). The UK National Lottery and the Arts: Reflections on the Lottery's impact and development. *International Journal of Arts Management, 3*(1), 19–31.

Danyluk, M., & Ley, D. (2007). Modalities of the new middle class: Ideology and behavior in the journey to work from gentrified neighbourhoods in Canada. *Urban Studies, 44*(11), 2195–2210.

Davidson, E. J. (2011). *The burdens of aspiration: Schools, youth, and success in the divided social worlds of Silicon Valley.* NYU Press.

Davies, B. (1999a). *From voluntryism to welfare state: A history of the youth service in England Volume 1, 1939–1979*. National Youth Agency.

Davies, B. (1999b). *From Thatcherism to New Labour: A history of the youth service in England Volume 2, 1979–1999*. National Youth Agency.

Davies, S., & Mehta, J. (2013). Educationalization. In J. Aninsworth (Ed.), *Sociology of education: An A-to-Z guide* (pp. 228–230). SAGE.

Dell, C. A. (2015). *Young offender legislation in Canada: A commentary*. Correctional Service Canada. www.csc-scc.gc.ca/research/forum/e112/e112k-eng.shtml

DeLuca, S., Clampet-Lundquist, S., & Edin, K. (2016). *Coming of age in the other America*. Russell Sage Foundation.

Department for Culture, Media and Sport. (1999). *The contribution arts and sport can make*. Policy Action Team 10, HMSO.

Department for Education and Skills. (2006). *The London Challenge*. http://webarchive. nationalarchives.gov.uk/20070101091332/http://www.dfes.gov.uk/londonchallenge

Dewdney, A., & Lister, M. (1988). *Youth, culture and photography (Youth Questions)*. Palgrave Macmillan.

DiGiacomo, D., & Gutiérrez, K. D. (2015). Relational equity as a design tool within making and tinkering activities. *Mind, Culture, and Activity*, 22(1), 1–15.

Dillabough, J.-A., & Kennelly, J. (2010). *Lost youth in the global city: Class, culture, and the urban imaginary*. Routledge.

Dorling, D. (2011). *Injustice: Why social inequality persists*. Policy Press.

Douglas, S. (1991). Introduction. In S. Douglas (Ed.), *Vancouver anthology: The institutional politics of art* (pp. 11–22). Talonbooks.

Druick, Z. (2007). *Projecting Canada: Government policy and documentary film at the National Film Board*. McGill-Queen's University Press.

Duffy, M. (2011). *Making care count: A century of gender, race, and paid care work*. Rutgers University Press.

Duxbury, N., Garrett-Petts, W., & McLennan, D. (2015). *Cultural mapping as cultural enquiry*. Routledge.

Edwards, A. (2011). Building common knowledge at the boundaries between professional practices: Relational agency and relational expertise in systems of distributed expertise. *International Journal of Educational Research*, 50(1), 33–39.

Erstad, O., Gile, O., Sefton-Green, J., & Arnseth, H. C. (2016). *Learning identities, education and community: Young lives in the cosmopolitan city*. Cambridge University Press.

Evans, G., & Foord, J. (2008). Cultural mapping and sustainable communities: Planning for the arts revisited. *Cultural Trends*, 17(2), 65–96.

Fernandez, S., & Fraticelli, R. (1994) *Culture force*. Toronto Arts Council.

Ferreira, V. S. (2016). Aesthetics of youth scenes: From arts of resistance to arts of existence. *YOUNG*, 24(1), 66–81.

Field, J. (2006). *Lifelong learning and the new educational order* (New rev. ed.). Trentham Books.

Field, J. (2008). *Social capital (Key Ideas)*. Routledge.

Filewod, A. D. (2011). *Committing theatre: Theatre radicalism and political intervention in Canada*. Between the Lines.

Firmstone, J., Georgiou, M., Husband, C., Marinkova, M., & Steibel, F. (2019). *Representations of minorities in the media: UK, final analysis report*. University of Leeds.

Fitzsimmons Frey, H., & Kerekes, J. (2021). Physical culture drills and Alberta girls stepping together across time. *Girlhood Studies, 14*(3). https://doi.org/10.3167/ghs.2021.140308

Flicker, S., Danforth, J. Y., Wilson, C., Oliver, V., Larkin, J., Restoule, J. P., Mitchell, C., Konsmo, E., Jackson, R., & Prentice, J. (2014). "Because we have really unique art": Decolonizing research with Indigenous youth using the arts. *International Journal of Indigenous Health, 10*(1), 16–34.

Florida, R. (2002). *The rise of the creative class: And how it's transforming work, leisure, community and everyday life.* Basic Books.

Floridi, L. (2014). *The fourth revolution: How the infosphere is reshaping human reality.* Oxford University Press.

Fornas, J., Lindberg, U., & Sernhede, O. (1995). *In Garageland: Rock, youth and modernity.* Routledge.

Freire, P. (2000). *Pedagogy of the oppressed* (M. B. Ramos, Trans.). Continuum.

Freire, P. (2015). *Pedagogy of the oppressed* (30th anniversary ed.). Bloomsbury.

Furlong, A., & Cartmel, F. (2006). *Young people and social change: New perspectives* (2nd ed.). Open University Press.

Gallagher, K. (2014). *Why theatre matters: Urban youth, engagement, and a pedagogy of the real.* University of Toronto Press.

Gallagher, K., Rodricks, D. J., & Jacobson, K. (Eds.). (2020). *Global youth citizenry and radical hope: Enacting community-engaged research through performative methodologies.* Springer.

Garnham, N. (1987). Concepts of culture: Public policy and the cultural industries. *Cultural Studies, 1,* 23–27.

Garnham, N. (2005). From cultural to creative industries: An analysis of the implications of the "creative industries" approach to arts and media policy making in the United Kingdom. *International Journal of Cultural Policy, 11,* 15–29.

Gerrard, J. (2014). Counter-narratives of educational excellence: Free schools, success, and community-based schooling. *British Journal of Sociology of Education, 35*(6), 876–894.

Gerrard, J. (2016). *Radical childhoods: Schooling and the struggle for social change.* Manchester University Press.

Gilborn, D. G. (2013). Interest-divergence and the colour of cutbacks: Race, recession and the undeclared war on Black children. *Discourse, 34*(4), 477–491. https://doi.org/10.1080/01596306.2013.822616

Gilje, O. (2012). Trajectories and timescales: The stories of four young Scandinavian filmmakers. In O. Erstad & J. Sefton-Green (Eds.), *Learning lives: Transactions, technologies, and learner identity* (pp. 198–214). Cambridge University Press.

Gilje, O., & Groeng, L. (2015). The making of a filmmaker: Curating learning identities in early careers. *E-Learning and Digital Media, 12*(2), 212–225. https://doi.org/10.1177/2042753014568177

Glaser, B., & Strauss, A. (1967). *The discovery of grounded theory.* Aldine de Gruyter.

Goldberg, D. T. (2009). *The threat of race: Reflections on racial neoliberalism.* Wiley-Blackwell.

Goldberg, D. T. (2012). When race disappears. *Comparative American Studies, 10*(2–3), 116–127.

Goldin, C., & Katz, L. (2008). *Race between education and technology.* Harvard University Press.

Gosetti-Ferencei, J. A. (2018). *The life of imagination: Revealing and making the world.* Columbia University Press.

Graham, P. (2001). Space: Irrealis objects in technology policy and their role in a new political economy. *Discourse & Society, 12*(6), 761–788. https://doi.org/10.1177/09579265 01012006003

Graham, S., & Marvin, S. (2001). *Splintering urbanism: Networked infrastructures, technological mobilities and the urban condition.* Routledge.

Greller, M. (2015). Leasehold: An institutional framework for understanding nonprofit governance in a civil society context. *Administrative Sciences, 5,* 165–176.

Griffin, C. (1993). *Representations of youth: The study of youth and adolescence in Britain and America (Feminist Perspectives).* Polity.

Grotowski, J. (1968). *Towards a poor theatre.* Simon & Schuster.

Groves, N. (2013, February 4). Arts head: Deborah Bestwick, director, Ovalhouse. *The Guardian.* https://www.theguardian.com/culture-professionals-network/culture-professionals-blog/2013/feb/04/deborah-bestwick-ovalhouse-theatre-interview

Hall, P. D. (1992). *Inventing the nonprofit sector and other essays in philanthropy, voluntarism, and nonprofit organizations.* Johns Hopkins University Press.

Hall, S. (2000). The multicultural question. In D. Morley (Ed.), *Stuart Hall: Selected writings, essential essays, Volume 2* (pp. 95–133). Duke University Press.

Hall, S. (2016). The rise and fall of urban regeneration policy in England, 1965 to 2015. In F. Weber & O. Kühne (Eds.), *Fraktale Metropolen. Hybride Metropolen* (pp. 313–330). Springer.

Hall, S., Massey, D., & Rustin, M. (2013). *After neoliberalism? The Kilburn Manifesto.* Lawrence & Wishart.

Hansman, G. (2016). Personalized learning: Back to the future? *Teacher, 28*(3). https://issuu. com/teachernewsmag/docs/2015_jan-feb_teacher_issuu/6

Hargraves, G. (2000). The review of vocational qualifications, 1985 to 1986: An analysis of its role in the development of competence-based vocational qualifications in England and Wales. *British Journal of Educational Studies, 48*(3), 285–308.

Hargreaves, A., & Fullan, M. (2012). *Professional capital: Transforming teaching in every school.* Routledge.

Harvey, D. (1989). *The condition of postmodernity: An enquiry in the origins of cultural change.* Blackwell.

Harvey, D. (2007). *A brief history of neoliberalism* (New ed.). Oxford University Press.

Harvey, D. (2011). *The enigma of capital and the crises of capitalism.* Profile Books.

Harvey, I., Skinner, M., & Parker, D. (2002). *Being seen, being heard: Young people and moving image production.* National Youth Agency/British Film Institute.

Heath, S. B. (2012). *Words at work and play: Three decades in family and community life.* Cambridge University Press.

Heath, S. B., & McLaughlin, M. W. (1993). *Identity and inner-city youth: Beyond ethnicity and gender.* Teachers College Press.

Heath, S. B., & Roach, A. (1999). Imaginative actuality: Learning in the arts during the non-school hours. In Arts Education Partnership (Ed.), *Champions of change: The impact of the arts on learning* (pp. 19–34). Arts Education Partnership & President's Committee on Arts and Humanities.

Heath, S. B., Soep, E., & Roach, A. (1998). *Living the arts through language + learning: A report on community based youth organizations*. National Assembly of State Arts Agencies.

Heathcote, D., Johnson, L., & O'Neill, C. (1984). *Dorothy Heathcote: Collected writings on education and drama*. Hutchinson.

Hebdige, D. (1979). *Subculture: The meaning of style*. Routledge.

Hesmondhalgh, D. (2012). *The cultural industries* (3d ed.). SAGE.

Hesmondhalgh, D., & Pratt, A. (2005). Cultural industries and cultural policy. *International Journal of Cultural Policy, 11*(1), 1–14.

Hill, A. (2021, January 3). Youth organisations in England face wholesale closure. *The Guardian*. https://www.theguardian.com/uk-news/2021/jan/03/youth-organisations-in-england-face-wholesale-closure

Himmelfarb, G. (1990). Victorian philanthropy: The case of Toynbee Hall. *The American Scholar, 59*(3), 373–384.

Hirsch, B. J. (2005). *A place to call home*. Teachers College Press.

Hitchins, G., Campbell, T., & Sefton-Green, J. (2014). *Now we are 10: Supporting Talent into Enterprise for London's creative sector, 2004 to 2014*. BOP Consulting.

Hochschild, A. (1983). *The managed heart: Commercialization of human feeling*. University of California Press.

Howkins, J. (2002). *The creative economy: How people make money from ideas*. Penguin.

Huq, R. (2003). Global youth cultures in localized spaces: The case of the new Asian dance music and French rap. In D. Muggleton & R. Weinzierl (Eds.), *The post-subcultures reader* (pp. 195–208). Berg.

Hutchings, M., Francis, B., & De Vries, R. (2017). *Chain effects: The impact of academy chains on low income students*. Sutton Trust.

Huxley, A. (1937). *Ends and means*. Harper & Brothers.

Hyland, T. (1996). National vocational qualifications, skills training and employers' needs: Beyond Beaumont and Dearing. *Journal of Vocational Education and Training, 48*(4), 349–365.

Hyndman, N., & McMahon, D. (2010). The evolution of the UK charity Statement of Recommended Practice: The influence of key stakeholders. *European Management Journal, 28*(6), 455–466. https://doi.org/10.1016/j.emj.2010.06.004

Idriss, S. (2017). *Young migrant identities: Creativity and masculinity*. Routledge.

Ilcan, S., & Basok, T. (2004). Community government: Voluntary agencies, social justice, and the responsibilization of citizens. *Citizenship Studies, 8*(2), 129–144. https://doi.org/10.1080/1362102042000214714

Ito, M., Baumer, S., Bittanti, M., boyd, d., Cody, R., Herr-Stephenson, B., Horst, H. A., Lange, P. G., Mahendran, D., Martínez, K. Z., Pascoe, C. J., Perkel, D., Robinson, L., Sims, C., & Tripp, L. (2010). *Hanging out, messing around, and geeking out: Kids living and learning with new media*. MIT Press.

Ito, M., Martin, C., Pfister, R. C., Rafalow, M. H., Salen, K., & Wortman, A. (2018). *Affinity online: How connection and shared interest fuel learning (Connected Youth and Digital Futures)*. NYU Press.

Izatt-White, M. (2011). Methodological crises and contextual solutions: An ethnomethodologically informed approach to understanding leadership. *Leadership, 7*(2), 119–135.

Jeffs, T., & Smith, M. (1987). *Youth work*. Macmillan.

Jeffs, T., & Smith, M. (2005). *Informal education: Conversation, democracy and learning.* Educational Heretics Press.

Jenkins, H., Shresthova, S., & Gamber-Thompson, L. (2016). *By any media necessary: The new youth activism (Connected Youth and Digital Futures).* NYU Press.

Jenson, J., & de Castell, S. (2010). Gender, simulation and gaming: Research review and redirections. *Simulation and Gaming, 41*(1), 51–71.

Jiwani, Y. (2006). *Discourses of denial: Mediations of race, gender and violence.* UBC Press.

Johnes, R. (2017). *Entries to arts subjects at Key Stage 4.* Education Policy Institute.

Jones, K., & Thomson, P. (2008). Policy rhetoric and the renovation of English schooling: The case of Creative Partnerships. *Journal of Education Policy, 23*(6), 715–727.

Judd, A. (2015, September 1). New curriculum launched for BC public schools. *Global News.* https://globalnews.ca/news/2196704/new-curriculum-launched-for-b-c-public-schools

Julian, E. A. (1992). Equity at Toronto Arts Council: A brief history. Toronto Arts Council. https://torontoartscouncil.org/reports-and-resources/toronto-arts-council-equity-framework/equity-at-toronto-arts-council-a-brief-history

Kapoor. N. (2013). The advancement of racial neoliberalism in Britain. *Ethnic and Racial Studies, 36*(6), 1028–1046.

Keck, J. M. (1995). *Making work: Federal job creation policy in the 1970s* (Doctoral dissertation]. University of Toronto.

Keller, J., & Ringrose, J. (2014). *Feminisms in schools: Young digital feminist activism and mediated intimacies* [Paper presentation]. Mediated Intimacies Symposium, London, England, July 17.

Kelly, O. (1984). *Community art and the state: Storming the citadels.* Comedia.

Kenway, J., & Bullen, E. A. (2007). The global corporate curriculum and the young cyberflaneur as global citizen. In N. Dolby & F. Rizvi (Eds.), *Youth moves: Identities and education in global perspective* (pp. 17–32). Routledge.

Kerr, L. A. (2011). *The educational production of students at risk* [Unpublished doctoral dissertation]. Ontario Institute for Studies in Education, University of Toronto.

Khan, N. (1976). *The arts Britain ignores: The arts of ethnic minorities in Britain.* Community Relations Commission.

Kirshner, B. (2015). *Youth activism in an era of education inequality.* NYU Press.

Kuppers, P. (2019). *Community performance: An introduction* (2nd ed.). Routledge.

Kwon, S. A. (2013). *Uncivil youth: Race, activism, and affirmative governmentality.* Duke University Press.

Ladwig, J. (2010). Beyond academic outcomes. *Review of Research in Education, 34,* 113–143.

Ladwig, J. (2018). Mapping the promise of non-schooled learning. In J. Sefton-Green & O. Erstad (Eds.), *Learning beyond the school: International perspectives on the schooled society* (pp. 79–86). Routledge.

Lambert, S. (2017). Public education: Reflections on fifteen years of public policy. *BC Studies, 194.*

Landry, C., Morley, D., Southwood, R., & Wright, P. (1985). *What a way to run a railroad: An analysis of radical failure.* Comedia.

Lang, S. (2012). *NGOs, civil society and the public sphere.* Cambridge University Press.

Lareau, A. (2011). *Unequal childhoods: Class, race, and family life, Second edition with an update a decade later* (2nd rev. ed.). University of California Press.

Lawrence, L. (2006). *Constructing success: The conundrum of evaluating a community-based program for street-involved youth* [Master's thesis]. Simon Fraser University.

Lefebvre, H. (1991). *The production of space* (D. Nicholson-Smith, Trans.). Blackwell.

Lemke, J., Lecusay, R., Cole, M., & Michalchik, V. (2015). *Documenting and assessing learning in informal and media-rich environments*. MIT Press.

Leslie, D., & Hunt, M. (2013). Securing the neoliberal city: Discourses of creativity and priority neighbourhoods in Toronto, Canada. *Urban Geography, 34*(8), 1171–1192.

Loyo, C. (2000). Fugitive events. A history of filmmaking in British Columbia, 1899–1970. In J. MacGregor (Ed.), *Cineworks Independent Filmmakers Society, 1980–2000* (pp. 86–120). Cineworks Independent Filmmakers Society.

Li, X. (2015). Ontario education governance 1995 to the present: More accountability, more regulation, and more centralization? *Journal of International Education & Leadership, 5*(1), 1–13.

Lindgren, A. (2017). Beyond primary sources: Using dance documentation to examine attitudes towards diversity in the Massey Commission (1949–1951). In H. Davis-Fisch (Ed.), *Canadian performance histories and historiographies* (pp. 141–160). Playwrights Canada Press.

Lupton, R., & Obolenskaya, P. (2013). *Labour's record on education: Policy, spending and outcomes 1997–2010*. CASE, London School of Economics and Political Science. http://sticerd.lse.ac.uk/dps/case/spcc/wp03.pdf

Maira, S., & Soep, E. (2005). *Youthscapes: The popular, the national, the global*. University of Pennsylvania Press.

Marcus, G. (2011). Multi-sited ethnography: Five or six things I know about it now. In S. Coleman & P. von Hellermann (Eds.), *Multi-sited ethnography: Problems and possibilities in the translocation of research methods* (pp. 16–32). Routledge.

Masters, C., & Anderson Eng, D. (2006, September 15). Get Out! Youth Legacy Program—Evaluation and next steps [Administrative report]. City of Vancouver.

Matarasso, F. C. (1996). *Defining values: Evaluating arts programmes*. The Social Impact of the Arts, Working Paper 1. Comedia.

McClanahan, W. S., & Hartmann, T. A. (2018, November). *Designing for engagement: The experiences of tweens in the Boys & Girls Clubs' Youth Arts Initiative*. Wallace Foundation.

McClintock, A. (1995). *Imperial leather: Race, gender and sexuality in the colonial contest*. Routledge.

McGregor, G., Mills, M., Riele, K. T., Baroutsis, A., & Hayes, D. (2017). *Re-imagining schooling for education: Socially just alternatives*. Palgrave Macmillan.

McLaughlin, M. W. (1999). *Community counts: How youth organizations matter for youth development*. Public Education Network.

McLaughlin, M. W. (2018). *You can't be what you can't see: The power of opportunity to change young lives*. Harvard Educational Publishing Group.

McLaughlin, M. W., Irby, M. A., & Langman, J. (1994). *Urban sanctuaries: Neighbourhood organizations in the lives and futures of inner-city youth*. Jossey-Bass.

McLaughlin, M. W., Scott, W. R., Deschenes, S. N., Hopkins, K. C., & Newman, A. R. (2009). *Between movement and establishment: Organizations advocating for youth*. Stanford University Press.

Mercer, C. (2006). Cultural planning for urban development and creative cities. *Political Science, 58*(1), 1–27.

Meyer, J. W., Boli, J., Thomas, G. M., & Ramirez, F. O. (1997). World society and the nation-state. *American Journal of Sociology, 103*(1), 144–181. https://doi.org/10.1086/231174

Miles, S., Pohl, A., Stauber, B., Walther, A., Banha, R. M. B., & Gomes, M. D. C. (2002). *Communities of youth: Cultural practice and informal learning.* Ashgate.

Mills, S., & Kraftl, P. (Eds.). (2014). *Informal education, childhood and youth: Geographies, histories, practices.* Palgrave Macmillan.

Mitchell, C., & Moletsane, R. (2018). *Disrupting shameful legacies.* Brill Sense.

Mitchell, K. (2004). *Crossing the neoliberal line: Pacific Rim migration and the metropolis.* Temple University Press.

Monnet, N., & Boukala, M. (2018). Urban trajectories and posturing: The place of children and teenagers in the makeup of the city. *Enfances, Familles, Générations, 30,* 1–29.

Morrison, R. (2006, February 3). The magic round about: A visionary philanthropist is making history in North London. *The Times.* https://www.thetimes.co.uk/article/the-magic-round-about-rrbmsx3wsws

MTM Consulting. (2016). *MTM Conference 2016—Downloads.* https://mtmconsulting.co.uk/mtm-conference-2016-presentations

Murawski, M. (2021). *Museums as agents of change: A guide to becoming a changemaker.* Rowman & Littlefield.

Murray, C., & Hutton, T. (2012). Vancouver: The enigmatic emerging cultural metropolis. In H. Anheier & Y. R. Isar (Eds.), *Cities, cultural policy and governance* (pp. 310–321). SAGE.

Nasir, N. S., Jones, A., & McLaughlin, M. (2011). School connectedness for students in low-income urban high schools. *Teachers College Record, 113*(8), 1755–1793.

National Advisory Committee on Creative and Cultural Education. (1999, May). All our futures: Creativity, culture and education. http://sirkenrobinson.com/pdf/allourfutures.pdf

Neelands, J., Belfiore, E., Firth, C., Hart, N., Perrin, L., Brock, S., Holdaway, D., & Woddis, J. (2015). Enriching Britain: Culture, creativity and growth. The *final report of the Warwick Commission on the future of cultural value.* University of Warwick.

Nissen, M. (2012). *The subjectivity of participation.* Palgrave Macmillan.

Nyssens, M., & Defourny, J. (2013). Social innovation, social economy and social enterprise: What can the European debate tell us? In F. Moulaert, D. MacCallum, A. Mehmood, & A. Hamdouch (Eds.), *International handbook on social innovation: Social innovation, collective action and transdisciplinary research* (pp. 40–52). Elgar.

Oasis Skateboard Factory. (2013, January 29). *Oasis Skateboard Factory pops up at the Baitshop.* Blog. https://oasisskateboardfactory.blogspot.com/2013/01/oasis-skateboard-factory-pops-up-at.html

O'Connor, J., & Wynne, D. (1996). *From the margins to the centre: Cultural consumption and production in the post-industrial city.* Routledge.

O'Connor, P. (1986). *The story of St. Christopher House, 1912–1984.* Toronto Association of Neighborhood Services.

Office of the Deputy Prime Minister. (2000). *Our towns and cities: The future—Full report.* HMSO.

O'Hear, S., & Sefton-Green, J. (2004). Creative "communities": How technology mediates social worlds. In D. Miell & K. Littleton (Eds.), *Collaborative creativity: Contemporary perspectives* (pp. 113–125). Free Association Press.

Oldenburg, R (1989). *The great good place*. Paragon.

Ontario Arts Council. (2016). *Framing community: A community engaged art workbook*.

Ostrower, F., & Stone, M. M. (2006). Boards of nonprofit organizations: Research trends, findings and prospects for future research. In W. Powell & R. Steinberg (Eds.), *The nonprofit sector: A research handbook* (2nd ed., pp. 612–628). Yale University Press.

Parkinson, M. (1989). The Thatcher government's urban policy, 1979–89. *The Town Planning Review, 60*(4), 421–440.

Parrio, A. (2010, July 24). I spent my 20s working with Toronto youth, and today's gun violence conversations feel like déja vu. *CBC Arts*. https://www.cbc.ca/arts/i-spent-my-20s-working-with-toronto-youth-and-today-s-gun-violence-conversations-feel-like-deja-vu-1.4759224

Parsons, C., Godfrey, R., Annan, G., Cornwall, J., Dussart, M., Hepburn, S., Howlett, K., & Wennerstrom, V. (2005). *Minority exclusions and the Race Relations (Amendment) Act 2000*. Department for Education and Skills.

Perreault, A. (2018, August 8). Wapikoni Mobile Trailer prepares Indigenous youth with empowerment and direction. *NetNewsLedger*. https://www.netnewsledger.com/2018/08/08/wapikoni-mobile-trailer-prepares-indigenous-youth-with-empowerment-and-direction

Phillips-Watts, K., Hampton, C., Tsang, A., Doubliard, J., & Barsanti, J. (2005). Gentrification in Vancouver: A study of changing urban dynamics. https://ibis.geog.ubc.ca/courses/geob479/classof05/gentrification/Vangents-What-is-Gentrification.htm

Piketty, T. (2020). *Capital and ideology*. Belknap.

Pollen, A. (2015). *Kindred of the Kibbo Kift*. Donlon.

Poyntz, S. R. (2008). *Producing publics: An ethnographic study of democratic practice and youth media production and mentorship* [Unpublished doctoral dissertation]. University of British Columbia.

Poyntz, S. R. (2017). Remediating democracy: Participatory youth media scenes, cultural friction and media reform. In B. De Abreu, P. Mihailidis, A. Lee, J. Melki, & J. McDougall (Eds.), *International handbook of media literacy* (pp. 159–173). Routledge.

Poyntz, S. R. (2018). Vancouver youthspaces: A political economy of digital learning communities. In M. Dezuanni, M. Foth, K. Mellan, & H. Hughes (Eds.), *Digital participation through social living labs: Valuing local knowledge, enhancing engagement* (pp. 277–297). Elsevier.

Poyntz, S. R. (2021). Producing authenticity: Urban youth arts, rogue archives and negotiating a home for social justice. Special section on "Youth and Social Media—From Vulnerability to Empowerment & Equality." *Studies in Social Justice, 15*(3), 375–396.

Poyntz, S. R., Coles, R., Fitzsimmons Frey, H., Bains, A., Sefton-Green, J., & Hoechsmann, M. (2019). The non-formal learning sector, youth provision and paradox in the learning city. *Oxford Review of Education, 45*(2), 258–278.

Preston, S. (2013). Managed hearts? Emotional labour and the applied theatre facilitator in urban settings. *Research in Drama Education, 18*(3), 230–245.

Puzio, A., & Valshtein, T. (2022). Gender segregation in culturally feminized work: Theory and evidence of boys' capacity for care. *Psychology of Men & Masculinities, 23*(3), 271–284. http://dx.doi.org/10.1037/men0000397

Ratnam, A., & Vasudevan, N. (2018). The personal and pedagogical in the 21st century: Experiments in learning about marriage. In J. Sefton-Green & O. Erstad (Eds.), *Learning beyond the school: International perspectives on the schooled society* (pp. 209–225). Routledge.

Razack, S. (2002). *Race, space, and the law: Unmapping a White settler society*. Between the Lines.

Rees, J. (2014). Public sector commissioning and the third sector: Old wine in new bottles. *Public Policy and Administration, 29*(1) 45–63.

Rennie, E. (2012). *Life of SYN: A story of the digital generation*. Monash University Publishing.

Rennie, E., & Podkalicka, A. M. (2014). Youth development or media innovation? The outcomes of youth media enterprise. *Communications & Media Studies, 7*(1), 98–110.

Rexe, D. (2015). Thawing the tuition freeze: The politics of policy change in comparative perspective. *Canadian Political Science Review, 9*(2), 79–111.

Robinson, D., & Keavy, M. (2016). *Arts of engagement: Taking aesthetic action in and beyond the Truth and Reconciliation Commission of Canada*. Wilfrid Laurier University Press.

Rose, N. (1999). *Governing the soul: Shaping of the private self*. Free Association Books.

Rowsell, J. (2012). *Working with multimodality: Rethinking literacy in a digital age*. Routledge.

Royal Commission on National Development in the Arts, Letters and Sciences. (1951). *Report: Royal Commission on National Development in the Arts, Letters and Sciences: 1949–1951*. King's Printer.

Russo, A. P., & van der Borg, J. (2010). An urban policy framework for culture-oriented economic development: Lessons from the Netherlands. *Urban Geography, 31*(5), 668–690.

Saha, A. (2018). *Race and the cultural industries*. Polity.

Salverson, J. (2011). *Community engaged theatre and performance*. Playwrights Canada Press.

Sandlin, J. A. (2009). *Handbook of public pedagogy: Education and learning beyond schooling* (Studies in Curriculum Theory Series). Routledge.

Scannell, P. (2014). *Television and the meaning of "live": An enquiry into the human condition*. Cambridge University Press.

Sefton-Green, J. (2008). What future for the non-formal learning sector? An *analytic review commissioned by the London Development Agency*. https://julianseftongreen.net/wp-content/uploads/2022/11/seftongreen_NFLS_essay.pdf

Sefton-Green, J. (2013). *Learning at not-school: A review of study, theory, and advocacy for education in non-formal settings*. MIT Press.

Sefton-Green, J. (2018). Outing the "out" in out-of-school: A comparative international perspective. In J. Sefton-Green & O. Erstad (Eds.), *Learning beyond the school: International perspectives on the schooled society* (pp. 193–208). Routledge.

Sefton-Green, J., & Erstad, O. (2018). *Learning beyond the school: International perspectives on the schooled society* (Routledge Research in Education). Routledge.

Sefton-Green, J., Thomson, P., Jones, K., & Bresler, L. (Eds.). (2011). *The Routledge international handbook of creative learning* (Routledge International Handbooks of Education). Routledge.

Sefton-Green, J., Watkins, S. C., & Kirshner, B. (2019). *Young people's transitions into creative work: Negotiating challenges and opportunities*. Routledge.

Selwyn, N. (2010). *Inspired by technology, driven by pedagogy: A systematic approach to technology-based school innovations*. CERI.

Sennett, R. (2017). The public realm. In S. Hall & R. Burdett (Eds.), *The SAGE handbook of the 21st century city* (pp. 585–601). SAGE.

Shaffeeullah, N. A. (2020). Radical mentorship and more: Community arts as a pathway to equity. *Canadian Theatre Review, 181*(1), 29–33. https://doi.org/10.3138/ctr.181.005

Shaffeeullah, N. A., Boulay, J., & Sarker, S. (2020). Manifesting the future. *Theatre Research in Canada, 41*(2), 278–282. https://doi.org/10.3138/tric.41.2.f01

Shaker, E., & Hennessey, T. (2018, June 21). Course correction: Fixing a flawed funding formula. *Education Forum.* https://education-forum.ca/2018/06/21/course-correction

Sieverts, T. (2003). *Cities without cities: Between place and world, space and time, town and country.* Routledge.

Sinker, R. (2000). Multimedia. In J. Sefton-Green & R. Sinker (Eds.), *Evaluating creativity making and learning by young people* (pp. 43–69). Routledge.

Smith, A. (1996). *The new urban frontier: Gentrification and the revanchist city.* Routledge.

Smith, A. (2005). *Conquest: Sexual violence and American Indian genocide.* South End Press.

Smith, C. (1998). *Creative Britain.* Faber & Faber.

Smithsimon, G. (2010). Inside the empire: Ethnography of a global citadel in New York. *Urban Studies, 47*(4), 699–724.

Soep, L., & Chavez, V. (2010). *Drop that knowledge: Youth radio stories.* University of California Press.

Soja, E. (1996). *Thirdspace: Journeys to Los Angeles and other real and imagined places.* Blackwell.

Standing, G. (2016). *The precariat: The new dangerous class* (Bloomsbury Revelations). Bloomsbury.

Standing Committee on Canadian Heritage. (1999). *Sense of place, a sense of being: The evolving role of the federal government in support of culture in Canada.* House of Commons, Canadian Parliament.

Standing Senate Committee on Aboriginal Peoples. (2011). *Reforming First Nations education: From crisis to hope.* Senate of Canada.

Stevenson, D., Balling, G., & Kann-Rasmussen, N. (2017). Cultural participation in Europe: Shared problem or shared problematisation? *International Journal of Cultural Policy, 23*(1), 89–106, doi:10.1080/10286632.2015.1043290

Stevie. (2017, August 4). *Almeida (the Glorious) (The AMY Project), 2017 SummerWorks review.* Mooney on Theatre Blog. https://www.mooneyontheatre.com/2017/08/04/almeida-the-glorious-the-amy-project-2017-summerworks-review

Straw, W. (1991). Systems of articulation, logics of change: Communities and scenes in popular music. *Cultural Studies, 5*(3), 368–388.

Sukarieh, M., & Tannock, S. (2015). *Youth rising? The politics of youth in the global economy.* Routledge.

Taucar, J. (2016). Acting out(side) the Canadian multicultural "script" in Toronto's ethnocultural festivals [Unpublished doctoral dissertation]. University of Toronto.

Threadgold, S. (2017). *Youth, class and everyday struggles.* Routledge.

Travlou, P. (2003). *Teenagers and public space: Literature review.* Edinburgh College of Art and Heriot-Watt University.https://www.openspace.eca.ed.ac.uk/wp-content/uploads/2015/10/Teenagers-and-Public-Space-literature-review.pdf

Trotter, L. D., & Mitchell, A. (2018). Academic drift in Canadian institutions of higher education: Research mandates, strategy, and culture. *Canadian Journal of Higher Education, 48*(2), 92–108.

Turner, F. (2008). *From counterculture to cyberculture: Stewart Brand, the Whole Earth Network, and the rise of digital utopianism.* University of Chicago Press.

Tyner, K. (2009). Mapping the field: Results of the 2008 survey of youth media organizations in the United States. *Youth Media Reporter, 3,* 107–143.

United Nations General Assembly. (1998). *International Decade for a Culture of Peace and Non-Violence for the Children of the World 2001–2010* (Session 53).

Urban Task Force. (1999). *Towards an urban renaissance.* Spon.

Vancouver City Council. (1991). *Vancouver central area plan: Goals and land use policy.* City of Vancouver Planning Department.

Vizenor, G. (1999). *Manifest manners: Narratives on post-Indian survivance.* University of Nebraska Press.

Wagner, A. (2015). Nonprofit governance, organizational purposiveness and design. *Administrative Sciences, 5*(4), 177–187.

Walford, G. (2014). From city technology colleges to free schools: Sponsoring new schools in England. *Research Papers in Education, 29*(3), 315–329.

Ward, C. (1978). *The child in the city.* Pantheon.

Warner, M. (2002). *Publics and counterpublics.* Zone Books.

Warner, R. (2006). Towards a new youth program/policy remix: Fresh arts and the case for community-based, youth urban arts programming. Prepared for the Ontario Region of the Department of Canadian Heritage.

Wasteneys, H. C. F. (1975). *A history of the University Settlement of Toronto 1910–1958: An exploration of the social objectives of the University Settlement and of their implementation* [Doctoral dissertation]. University of Toronto.

Watkins, C. S. (2019). *Don't knock the hustle: Young creatives, tech ingenuity, and the making of a new innovation economy.* Beacon Press.

Weber, M. (1947). *The theory of social and economic organization* (A. M. Henderson & T. Parsons, Trans.). Free Press.

Weiler, J., & Mohan, A. (2009). *Catalyst, collaborator, connector: The social innovation model of 2010 Legacies Now—Case study commissioned for the International Olympic Committee.* 2010 Legacies Now Corporation. www.2010andbeyond.ca/media/pdf/Catalyst_Collaborator_Connector_The_Social_Innovation_Model_of_2010_Legacies_Now.pdf

Werquin, P. (2010). *Recognition of formal and non-formal and informal learning: Outcomes, policies and country practices.* OECD Publishing.

Wilkinson, R., & Pickett, K. (2010). *The spirit level: Why equality is better for everyone.* Penguin.

Wingfield, A. H. (2009). Racializing the glass elevator: Reconsidering men's experiences with women's work. *Gender & Society, 23*(1), 5–26. https://doi.org/10.1177/0891243208323054

Wise, P. (2002). Cultural policy and multiplicities. *International Journal of Cultural Policy, 8*(2), 221–231.

Woddis, C. (2007, October 24). Peter Oliver: Pioneering spirit of young people's alternative theatre. *The Guardian*. www.theguardian.com/news/2007/oct/24/guardianobituaries. obituaries

Wright, R., John, L., Alaggia, R., & Sheel, J. (2006). Community-based arts program for youth in low-income communities: A multi-method evaluation. Child and Adolescent Social Work Journal, 23, 635–652. https://doi.org/10.1007/s10560-006-0079-0

Yerichuk, D. (2014). "Socialized music": Historical formations of community music through social rationales. *Action, Criticism, and Theory for Music Education*, 13(1), 126–154.

Other Documents

Christ Church (Oxford) United Clubs, 2005.

Monsoon Festival program (South Asian Arts).

Ovalhouse annual reports, 1978, 1984, 1992, 1994, 1995, 2005, 2017.

Ovalhouse brochure, 1979.

Paddington Arts 20th Anniversary Reunion, 1987–2007.

Paddington Arts Report into Performing Arts and Media, 2011.

Paddington Arts business plans, 1995, 2002–2005, 2006–2009.

Paddington Arts development plan, 1998–2001.

Paddington Arts annual reports, 2012–2013, 2016–2017.

Roundhouse annual reports, 2005, 2008, 2015.

SKETCH annual reports, 2005, 2010, 2020.

SKETCH initial notebook/fundraising document, 1996.

"Sketching a portrait," 2000, document in the SKETCH Archive.

The AMY Project Youth Feedback, 2018.

Unity Charity annual reports, 2013, 2014, 2015, 2017.

INDEX

For the benefit of digital users, indexed terms that span two pages (e.g., 52–53) may, on occasion, appear on only one of those pages.

Tables and figures are indicated by t and f following the page number